THE FACE OF LOVE

The Face of Love

Feminism and the Beauty Question

Ellen Zetzel Lambert

Beacon Press : Boston

Beacon Press
25 Beacon Street
Boston, Massachusetts 02108-2892
www.beacon.org

Beacon Press books
are published under the auspices of
the Unitarian Universalist Association of Congregations.

First digital-print edition 2001

Library of Congress Cataloging-in-Publication Data
Lambert, Ellen Zetzel, 1940–
The face of love : feminism and the beauty question / Ellen Zetzel Lambert.
p.   cm.
Includes bibliographical references and index.
ISBN 0-8070-6501-3
1. English fiction—Women authors—History and criticism.   2. American fiction—Women authors—
History and criticism.   3. Feminine beauty (Aesthetics) in literature.   4. Beauty, Personal, in literature.   5.
Body, Human, in literature.   6. Feminism in literature.   7. Women in literature.   8. Love in literature.   9.
Face in literature.   I. Title.
PR830.B4L36   1995
823.009´353—dc20   94-37969

This book is dedicated to the memory of my father

Louis Zetzel

whose love of beauty in women and beauty in all its earthly manifestations greatly enriched as well as complicated my own relationship to the beauty question, and who would have been proud had he lived to see his daughter complete this book.

Contents

Acknowledgments   ix

Preface   xi

1   The Beauty Myths   1

2   The Woman of Parts   23

3   Beauty and Identity: The Woman's Perspective   55

4   Charlotte Brontë:
    "As Small and as Plain as Myself"   95

5   George Eliot: The Beauty of Presence   128

6   Two Mastectomy Narratives:
    Beauty and Body-Integrity   150

7   The Beauty of Age   181

Notes   205

Index   231

Acknowledgments

I want particularly to thank:

Mark Lambert, for saying, "You really should do something more with that allusion to the 'prettier-but-not-really-prettier-sister motif' in Victorian literature" — at a time when neither of us knew where that "something more" might take me.

The National Endowment for the Humanities, for enabling me to spend a year working on an earlier, more academic version of this book.

Morris Dickstein, Patricia Meyer Spacks, Toni Burbank, Rachel Brownstein, Marie Borroff, and Mary Jacobus — whose careful readings, criticism, and encouragement in the early stages of my work on this manuscript sustained me when I needed it most.

Judith Zetzel Nathanson, my sister, alter ego, and best of readers.

Alan Petraske, whose enthusiasm for the work and for me helped me find the right direction.

Martin Tesher, physician and friend.

M. Jeanne Smith, who helped me work through many of the personal issues dealt with in these pages and who has been one of my most important role models, not only on the beauty question.

Marya Van't Hul at Beacon Press, a wonderful editor, as patient as she is prompt, who always said enough but never too much — all skills which I, as a teacher of writing, know how to value.

Finally, in the end, for lightening the load (checking the references, cooking the meals) and altogether brightening my life, David Buxenbaum.

Preface

What is the nature of that elusive but surely real relation between a person's outward appearance and his or her inner nature? Why should some people seem so beautiful to us on a first meeting and then not beautiful as we come to know them better, while the beauty of others reveals itself to us only over time? And why is it that when we know ourselves loved by another we feel our whole aspect must be radically altered, so that we may ask ourselves with a mixture of wonder and delight, like the girl in the song from *West Side Story*,

> *"See the pretty girl in that mirror there!*
> *Who can that attractive girl be?*
> *Such a pretty face,*
> *Such a pretty dress,*
> *Such a pretty smile,*
> *Such a pretty me!"*

Personally, the beauty question seems always to have been a difficult one for me. I know that it matters to me how I look. I know my feelings about my appearance are highly unstable: I can feel amazed at my prettiness one moment and confirmed in the knowledge of my ugliness the next. And I know this is a subject that I'm not — or have not been — comfortable talking about. As a committed feminist, I've felt embarrassed that the beauty question *should* still matter to me. For we have been taught and I have believed that women's traditional concern for their appearances was a part, and perhaps the most pernicious part, of the patriarchal legacy that demanded a woman's subordination of her own self to masculine imperatives. The beauty question (we've been told) is not really a woman's question, or problem, at all but a man's question: it's just one of the ways in which men have forced women to define themselves in terms of their desirability to others.

And yet this dismissal has never felt quite right to me; it has seemed a little too easy. For the beauty question, the question of appearances, is *my* issue too, is *our* issue as women, is indeed *anyone's* issue as a human being. For the question of who one is on the outside is intimately bound up with who one is on the inside; appearances are a very part of our identity. So I can't, finally, accept the notion that the desire to please another person by our appearance is, by definition, to lessen, or imperil, our sense of ourselves. Jane Eyre, dressing herself on the morning of her first day at Thornfield, wanting to look her best, and reflecting on her persistent anxiety about her appearance, asks herself, as I have often asked myself: "And why had I these aspirations and these regrets?" And she answers herself, "It would be difficult to say: I could not then distinctly say it to myself; yet I had a reason, and a logical, natural reason too." Logical and natural, yes; and also difficult to explain, even to oneself. This book is an effort to explore the question Jane opens up for us here — Jane's question and my own question.

I don't think I'm alone among contemporary feminists in feeling that we have short-changed or oversimplified the question of appearances, and made taboo an issue that deserves to be explored in an open, nonjudgmental context. Sometimes at feminist gatherings, as well as in more intimate conversations with friends, I have felt the beauty question hovering in the air around us, like a guilty secret — or like a secret that, if "confessed," must quickly be exorcised. "Well, of course, we shouldn't care about these superficial, silly things; it's so ridiculously vain, and yet . . ." Then nervous laughter, relief, and on to more serious concerns — like sex. For sex, interestingly, is not a taboo subject for us today in the way that beauty is.

But if I found that I couldn't justify to myself my own incorrigible "vanity" and I couldn't find a way to talk seriously about the beauty question with other women, I discovered that, as a reader of fiction as well as a teacher and critic of literature, I could enter into the lives of fictive women where the beauty question was sometimes addressed more seriously — or at least honored, as Jane Eyre honors it. To be sure, I didn't set out to pursue the beauty question in my reading. But we compulsive readers of fiction are always, consciously or unconsciously, searching for ways to resolve or gain insight into issues which perplex us in our own lives. In some major women's novels of the late eighteenth and nineteenth centuries the beauty question does get addressed — not as an issue which is simply assumed to be important, as a heroine might be assumed to be beautiful, but precisely as the beauty question felt to me in my own life: as a *problematic* issue. And I found that a number of earlier women novelists had found (if not always without difficulty) a way of valuing appearances in their fictions — and perhaps also in their lives — that was not destructive to a woman's self-esteem. If hesitant to talk about the issue of appearances on a personal level, I felt perfectly free to contemplate it and eventually to write about it, at this "safe" remove: how did English women writers in the late eighteenth and nineteenth centuries, at a time when women writers were for the first time writing novels for a largely female audience, deal with the beauty question in presenting their heroines? That was a question I could ask. And with that question in mind, I began writing this book. In the fictions of women novelists of that earlier period I discovered a model. And at some point in the writing of this book I decided that I wanted my own personal struggle with the beauty question, at various stages in my life, to be part of the story too — hoping that my own narrative might strike a resonant chord, and perhaps be helpful to readers struggling with various aspects of the beauty question in various stages of their own lives.

However, it was not until most of the material that appears in the following pages was written, that I suddenly realized just how deeply rooted was that personal part of it for me. It began for me, like so many of our life issues, in the experience of early childhood.

THE FACE OF LOVE

CHAPTER 1

The Beauty Myths

*A*t various times over the years I have been moved to look through the photographs of my early childhood that are gathered together in what we then called my "baby book." The pale blue satin cover is faded now almost to white, and the ribbons which once held the pages in place are gone. But at some point (was it in my early adolescence?) I arranged the pages in sequence as best I could. On the upper right corner of the flyleaf, neatly inked in my mother's hand, is *Ellen.* On the frontispiece, inside a garland of flowers, are inscribed the words "PRECIOUS MOMENTS: From Babyhood Through Childhood." The copyright date is 1939 (a year before my birth), and the opening thirty or so pages are devoted to the solemn record-keeping characteristic of child rearing in the 1940s. The dates at which I first sat up, took my first step, spoke my first word, got each new tooth, and, of course, was toilet-trained both by day (eighteen months!) and by night, are all duly recorded in their designated spaces. So are first excursions, and here the blank spaces allow some room for my mother's informal annotations — viz: "by car," *to Woolfinsohn's — liked riding but not being left alone;* "by boat," *Swan boat — Public Garden, with her Daddy;* "First long trip," *to Mt. Vernon, April 11, 1941, for Passover. Had a wonderful time!* The pages allotted to the events of each birthday give me glimpses of the growth of a child wonderfully at home in her world, exploring it for the most part earnestly, but also at times jubilantly.

Perhaps what most pleases me in these pages are glimpses they give of a loving mother, who took the time to fill each inch of available space with notations: *a nice day at home with her mother and*

1

Daddy, Grandma phoned from Mt. Vernon but E. wouldn't talk to her on the phone (on my first birthday); *ice cream and birthday cake, lots of callers, gave her a bicycle — loved it* (my second); and a few years later, when my father was stationed at a medical base in Texas during the war: *party at home in Leesville with seven little friends and several big ones . . . the first party to have real significance for E!* The notation for my sixth birthday says simply: *Out to lunch with a friend; dinner at night with Cele and Mac here. E enjoyed her day.* And there her record-keeping stops. My mother died of a rare and rapidly spreading form of cancer the following summer, two months before my seventh birthday. I notice, in my own awkward script, a few brief notations for two later years: for my eleventh birthday — *Hallowe'en Party*, and for my twelfth — *Theater party, 'Pirates of Penzance.'* By then I had a stepmother; again there were birthday parties that might be chronicled. But in those later childhood and adolescent years my baby book became my own private, even secret, treasure, the record of a lost, precious time — not a thing to be shared, not something to be publicly maintained, any more than (it seemed) my mother herself could be "kept alive" through shared memories, or even really acknowledged in the family at all.

Until I had a child of my own, the initial record-keeping section of the baby book held little interest for me. But in my later childhood and adolescent years I was drawn back again and again to the pages of photographs which make up the latter and longer section of my baby book. I was trying, no doubt, to "hold on to" the image of my lost mother, but also to hold on to the image of myself that I saw in these pictures: myself as a happy child, a loved child, a beautiful child. And still today, when I look through the pages of these snapshots (mostly black and white, with a few in radiant color from the later years), I am struck with wonder and delight by the beauty of the image of myself I see in them. Or by the image of *us*.

In one of the first photos, taken of me at the age of three months, I see my infant self resting lightly against my mother's chest. The fingers of her large hand reach around my back and arm to hold me against her body in sure support. Part of the beauty of this portrait depends upon the way the images of our two bodies echo one another, both in form and feeling. Our faces, each slightly turned toward the other, are both half shadowed. The tousled upsweep of my short dark hair repeats the curve of the neater upsweep of her comb-held plaits. The light, coming from the upper right, binds us together, as it first brightens the side of her hair and face, then touches my broad forehead, next my rounded cheek, the little dip of the mouth, and finally the tiny chin. My gaze turns outward, toward the world, and the grave tenderness I see in my own face seems a reflection of the expression in hers, as she gazes more knowingly yet equally trustingly, outward toward the camera's eye.

When I look through this baby book I also frequently return to a sequence of snapshots taken in June of 1942 when I was not quite two. The first shows me, with fair, wavy hair, dressed in a summer sunsuit, walking down the front steps of our apartment building, one hand holding the railing, the other not quite touching an outstretched arm (my mother's, there if needed). Then I'm at the bottom of the steps and up in her arms. Next I am pulling her *my* way, along the path that led toward the gate and the street beyond. Finally, I'm alone on the sidewalk. My hands are raised up and back over my head, my smile is ecstatic. I stretch one foot forward. I am sauntering, almost strutting, in my pride.

At the age of three I acquire what has to be called a dazzling smile. A color photo from this period shows blond hair cut round my face, one longer piece on the side, secured by a barrette, curving jauntily forward. At four I have become wistful, dreamy-eyed. In one picture, I look up through partly veiled lids, self-consciously, a half-smile on my lips. I remember how I loved the white pinafore with little eyelet holes and red trim at the edges I'm wearing in this picture. My sister, Judy, a year and a half younger than me, had its twin. In another photo from this period we're both in our pinafores, posing for the camera, me with my arm around her shoulder, holding down the ruffle of her pinafore, while the wind blows the sides of my own out like wings around me. Mine is the protective, slightly condescending "big sister smile"; Judy's is her famous "monkey-face" delighted (and delightful) grin. At six my hair is longer, and the coiffure has become more elaborate: a part in the middle, and on each side the front hair braided, drawn up, and joined with a small tie in the back. But I myself have become less demure. I see more images of myself in rapid action now — swinging up in the air, running with my hair flying out behind, swimming with our Mt. Vernon cousins in the striped, two-piece bathing suits which (like other presents from the various members of my mother's large family) came in threes for the three girl cousins: blue for me, pink for Judy, and yellow for our cousin Debbie.

There's a photo from this same summer of Judy and me, both beautiful, happy children, smiling as we snuggle on either side of my father, each claiming a seat on one of his knees, and all three of us squeezed into the large lounge chair in the backyard of the Mt. Vernon house. There is no photograph from the afternoon late that same summer when my father, reclining in this same chair, called me over to him to tell me my mother "would not be coming back to us anymore." "Where is she then?" "In heaven," he replied simply, as I stood there, not nestled in the chair with him that time but standing silently alongside it. And then, as I remember it, he asked me to go fetch Judy from her play at the swing-set so he could tell her too. "It's because of M-u-r-i-e-l," said my grandmother later that same afternoon, as the grown-ups stood over me and handed me the glass of water with which to swallow the aspirin for my headache. "But you're forgetting, Grandma," I thought to myself, "I know how to spell; I know what this is all about." Though of course I didn't, really. And very little was said out loud. We had been sent to Mt. Vernon to stay with our cousins that summer, my father just coming down for weekends. But being with my cousins, my aunt, and my grandmother for the summer months (though usually in a rented house in the country, where we swam and played together and the men — the fathers and my grandfather — came for weekends) was part of the familiar pattern of my early childhood, except that this summer, of course, my mother wasn't with us.

Sometime late in the spring she'd gotten sick; we were told she would have to go to the hospital for a little while. I watched while she packed a few things in a bag. Once Judy and I were taken to visit her in the hospital; she smiled at us from a bed in a small white room and showed me how to turn the crank that would make the front of the bed go up.

When the three of us came back home at the end of the summer to the apartment in Cambridge, a small, dark-haired woman was kneeling by the fireplace, vigorously polishing the andirons. Miss Oberacker had been a governess in her previous places of employment; she was coming to us out of "kindness," by courtesy of some wealthy friends of my father. And "Ocky," as we came to call her during her two-year interregnum, was fond of telling us stories of her better days, with better children — or at least with a better child. Judy, at five, was still cute and cuddly, numb perhaps in her uncomprehending grief, and Ocky petted her. But I was not cute: I was sullen, withdrawn. I told my father I didn't like Miss Oberacker and she couldn't tell me what to do because she wasn't my mother; but he just said he was sorry, he couldn't do anything about it. In the evening he sat in his chair in the living room and his face got red. I asked him what he was thinking about and he said, "You know what I'm thinking about." My second-grade teacher accused me of cheating on a homework assignment and grasped my arm hard in her hand. Once during "show and tell" I told my classmates our dog Terry had given birth to puppies and if anyone would like to have one, they should call my father. (A year or so earlier Terry had in fact had puppies, and one of the happiest memories of my childhood was of Judy, my mother, and me watching the puppies being born.) I couldn't explain to my father, when the parent of a classmate called to inquire about the puppies. I couldn't explain any of it to myself.

After my mother's death the pictorial as well as the narrative chronicle of my childhood ends. But there are two snapshots that someone — most likely me — pasted onto the next, waiting page of the baby book. They both must have been taken at the very end of that first summer back home in the Cambridge apartment. In one, my father, and sister, and I are sitting on the front porch steps of someone else's house (probably friends of my father). My father's face shows his deep sadness. He has one arm around Judy's shoulders, and she smiles blankly out at the camera. This is not the "monkey face" grin of former years; it is the empty smile of a child who does not know what has hit her. My whole body in this photo, on the other hand, speaks vividly of pain and withdrawal. I am sitting slightly behind my father's other shoulder, my body partly obscured, as if I'd refused to enter the circle offered by his other arm, which lies awkwardly in his lap. My legs are oddly askew. My long hair hangs in a plain line down one side of my face, and the expression on the face is guarded, neutral. In the other picture, my sister and I are sitting on another friend's front porch. My father has disappeared and my anger is more evident. Here I am scowling up at the camera, with lower lip protruding and hair unkempt. My posture is an exaggerated version of that in the first photo — legs drawn tightly together at the knees but thrust out at the calf, and here the feet are not curled inward. One foot protrudes as though I were about to kick something. My arms are stiffly braced by my sides. Judy sits at some distance from me, her hands clasped together in her lap, looking toward me perhaps in fear.

These last two photographs are not, as I read them, pictures of a pretty child in an unhappy time or a belligerent frame of mind. The child I see is an ugly child, who looks as though, even if she were smiling, her underlying sadness would still "show through." It would show up as awkwardness, a lack of harmony in the features themselves. The few scattered photos I've collected from my later childhood years confirm my sense that as I got older I got uglier, right up through adolescence. My face was too thin, my eyes too close together, my nose too long, my breasts (when they came) too small, my hips too large. And, particularly compared to the small-boned, delicate-featured stepmother who replaced Ocky after my father's two years of solitude, I was altogether too big and bony. The list of my physical defects was long and (as old diaries confirm) minutely inventoried by me, from top to toe. But it all added up to my sense of myself as graceless, undesirable, ugly. I felt that, compared with other girls I knew, I hadn't been blessed with good looks; I didn't have the "right" features, didn't "measure up."

Over the years I've lamented and wondered at the fact that I turned from such a pretty little child into such an unattractive girl. It is only now, in writing this book, that I am able to see that metamorphosis in different, and I believe in truer, terms. I understand now that the transformation of myself from a beautiful child to an ugly one is so distressing to me because deep down I have known all along what it was: neither an accident nor the fulfillment of an inevitable destiny but a response to an overwhelming loss. When I look at those early photos of myself I realize that what I am seeing and responding to so positively is the way delight and security inform a child's whole physical aspect. Looking at the photographs closely, I realize how many of the details I read as "beauty" can be referred back to the love at the center of that charmed circle. The aesthetically pleasing doubling of lines in that first photo has its source in a reciprocity of love between two people; the radiant smile on my face a few years later speaks to me of love; the two little braids on either side of my head, of attention paid; and all those outward-reaching, confident gestures, of a body at peace with itself in the world. And so it comes to me now, with the same rush of understanding, that what I am responding to, when I look at the images of myself sitting awkwardly on someone else's porch, with the wrong dress and the wrong hairstyle, and features which seem to have lost their right relation to one another, is the enormity of the loss that wrought such a change. And how could the very features of my face not look "wrong" when, in the most fundamental way possible, my whole life had gone wrong? I didn't just *become* ugly; my ugliness in those later childhood years was a response — in a sense *the most powerful response* I could make — to the turning upside down of my whole life.

Toni Morrison writes about a child's beauty or ugliness in the terms I am talking about here in her novel *The Bluest Eye*, but she places that vision in a larger, cultural context rather than a personal one,

where its effect — from the point of view of the unloved, unbeautiful child — is all the more devastating. The "adopted" ugliness of
the Breedloves, a black family living at the very bottom of the social scale in a small southern town in the 1940s, tells the same story
of sadness and self-contempt I see in the photos of my later childhood years.

> No one could have convinced them that they were not relentlessly
> and aggressively ugly. Except for the father, Cholly, whose ugli-
> ness (the result of despair, dissipation, and violence directed toward
> petty things and weak people) was behavior, the rest of the family
> — Mrs. Breedlove, Sammy Breedlove, and Pecola Breedlove —
> wore their ugliness, put it on, so to speak, although it did not be-
> long to them. The eyes, the small eyes set closely together under
> narrow foreheads. The low, irregular hairlines, which seemed even
> more irregular in contrast to the straight, heavy eyebrows which
> nearly met. Keen but crooked noses, with insolent nostrils. They
> had high cheekbones, and their ears turned forward. Shapely lips
> which called attention not to themselves but to the rest of the face.
> You looked at them and wondered why they were so ugly; you
> looked closely and could not find the source. Then you realized that
> it came from conviction, their conviction. It was as though some
> mysterious all-knowing master had given each one a cloak of ug-
> liness to wear, and they had each accepted it without question. The
> master had said, "You are ugly people." They had looked about
> themselves and saw nothing to contradict the statement; saw, in
> fact, support for it leaning at them from every billboard, every
> movie, every glance. "Yes," they had said. "You are right."[1]

Morrison's description makes it clear that the ugliness of the
Breedlove family is something at once subjectively true and objectively real: it is what anyone looking at them takes in. In some other
setting the Breedloves' "shapely lips" might have been the features
which called attention to themselves and sent a message of beauty
to the world. In this world, however, the observer sees what I see
when I look at the photos of my later childhood — irregularity,
wrongness; here — uneven hairlines, crooked noses, eyes too close

together. Yet these "ugly" features are the ones we register because they are the ones the Breedloves have *chosen* to give out. The Breedloves' ugliness, like mine as an ugly child, comes "from conviction, their conviction." They "wear" their ugliness, Morrison says, "put it on, . . . although it did not belong to them."

But if the Breedloves have "put on" their cloak of ugliness, they are no freer to take it off than I was after my mother's death — actually less so. For the cause of their ugliness is not the accidental loss of a nurturing mother but the willed hostility of a dominant white society, which relentlessly and continually reinforces their conviction. And it is Pecola's special tragedy that the cloak of ugliness is put upon her not only by the dominant white culture but by the members of her own family. Pecola cannot even imagine herself as a truly beautiful child. All she can do is long to be beautiful on the terms of the "all-knowing master," long for the bluest eye. If she could only *know herself* as beautiful, Morrison suggests, Pecola would *be* beautiful. But "thrown, in this way," Morrison says, "into the binding conviction that only a miracle could relieve her, she would never know her beauty. She would see only what there was to see: the eyes of other people" (p. 40). Pecola cannot see herself as beautiful because she cannot see herself as lovable. How could she, never having known love? Toward the end of the novel Morrison's narrator offers us a metaphor for the unrealized beauty of Pecola in her description of the "ugly" baby to which Pecola (made pregnant by her father's rape) might have given birth: "I thought about the baby that everybody wanted dead, and saw it very clearly. It was in a dark, wet place, its head covered with great O's of wool, the black face holding, like nickels, two clean black eyes, the flared nose, kissing-thick lips, and the living, breathing silk of black skin" (p. 148).

Here, Morrison allows the reader to see what Pecola cannot see in herself and in her world, and to know both as intrinsically lovable. She shows us the beautiful, imagined face of Pecola's unborn child with loving wonderment, and allows us to see as beautiful the very same features which call attention to themselves as "ugly" in the earlier passage. In fiction, the novelist can be the loving mother who confers on her creation the aspect of beauty, but in the "real" world of the novel this beautiful child is stillborn, for Pecola cannot love her child any more than she can love herself. It was easier for me as a young girl, I realize. My image of myself as an ugly child was not continuously, overwhelmingly reinforced as Pecola's is. And perhaps even more importantly, unlike her, as an adolescent I had the memory of a beautiful self to hold on to, and perhaps some-day to recover.

This book is written in defense of appearances, and our concern for our own appearances. But appearances seen not as an appendage to the self but as the very expression of the self—a self informed by the knowledge of its essential lovability. Or, beauty as the face of love. That's an eloquent phrase for me. It is, I discover looking back, my misremembering of a line from the final section of the Renaissance neoplatonic dialogue, *The Courtier*, by Baldesar Casti-glione, in which the oldest and wisest of a group of assembled courtiers defends men's love for a beautiful woman. Rhapsodically (and some might say sophistically) Bembo appeals to his fellow courtiers that they not "incur the wrath of God in speaking ill of beauty, which is a sacred thing." For, as he goes on to explain, "beauty springs from God and is like a circle, the center of which is goodness. And hence, as there can be no circle without a center, there can be no beauty without goodness." And Bembo defends a very debatable equation, which has been a crux of Western philos-ophy ever since Plato, between outer beauty and inner virtue.

> Thus, a wicked soul rarely inhabits a beautiful body, and for that reason outward beauty is a true sign of inner goodness. And this grace is impressed upon the body in varying degree as an index of the soul, by which it is outwardly known, as with trees in which the beauty of the blossoms is a token of the excellence of the fruit. The same is true of the human body, as we see from the physiogno-mists, who often discover in the face the character and sometimes the thoughts of men. . . . Hence, the ugly are also wicked, for the most part, and beautiful are good: and we may say that beauty is the

pleasant, cheerful, charming, and desirable face of the good, and that ugliness is the dark, disagreeable, unpleasant, and sorry face of evil.[2]

In linking Bembo's notion that the beauty of a woman's face is the highest human expression of the goodness of God's creation, and the idea that a child's knowledge of her beauty is dependent on her knowledge of her mother's love, I may seem to have made an unwarranted leap. But I think that Bembo and I are really saying essentially the same thing about appearances: that beauty is the outward expression of an inner harmony, whatever the source of that harmony. My beauty before my mother's death was indeed "the pleasant, cheerful, charming, and desirable face of the good"; and I think it is true to say that, though I was not ultimately myself the *cause* for its being so, my ugliness after her death was, like that of the Breedloves, a kind of evil: "dark, disagreeable, unpleasant, and sorry."

To define beauty as the face of love is, then, to make two related but distinct assertions. It is to say, first of all, that our *perception* of beauty is subjectively determined. My mother saw me as beautiful because she loved me; Castiglione's courtier sees a woman's face as beautiful because he loves her; the white society sees the Breedloves as ugly because they hate them. "The face of love" in this sense is the face seen by the lover. Or, as the maxim has it, "beauty is in the eye of the beholder." But to say that beauty is the face of love is also to affirm that the beautiful face is the one itself informed, or animated, *by* love. Thus as a small child I gave back to the world the reflection of the love I had received, and in so doing I was beautiful. The beautiful woman in *The Courtier* is beautiful because her acts are informed by goodness, ultimately by the spirit of her Creator which moves within her. And, like my own childhood ugliness, the ugliness of the Breedloves is the expression of their own self-hatred. In this second, and more fundamental sense, "the face of love" is the face of one who loves. We need not, then, wait upon the lover to pronounce our beauty; we are, so to speak, the custodians of our own beauty, as our appearance (whether or not anyone is there to see it) is the expression of our identity. And if we can change our feelings about ourselves (as I eventually did, and as the narrator, if not Pecola, does in *The Bluest Eye*), then we can change our appearances. To see beauty as the face of love rather than the arbitrary gift of fortune is, then, to enlarge our sense of life's possibilities. A beautiful child (or woman) can become the ugly child; but an ugly woman (or man) can also become a beautiful one.

For most of us the beauty question is not complicated, as for Morrison's Pecola, by the enormous issue of race in our culture. And my own status as an ugly child, being determined as it was by the misfortune of my mother's early death, is atypical in a different sense. And yet, as I look around me, at women of all ages, I see enormous insecurity about beauty in our culture. If most of the women I know are not convinced of their ugliness in the way I was as a child, they are acutely uncomfortable about the beauty question as it pertains to their own persons. My own unusual childhood experience, rather than being simply anomalous, would seem to have sensitized me to an anxiety about personal appearances which pervades women in our society generally.

Why should that be? I think the answer is not hard to find. The voices all around us, voices we hear every day on the street and in the marketplace, in every advertisement addressed to the female consumer and on every T.V. sit-com, do not send out the message that beauty is the face of love. On the contrary, what they tell us is that beauty is a way of *capturing* love. Beauty is not inwardly determined and hence contingent; it is outwardly fixed. "But," this voice continues, "if you've not been blessed with beauty, or have lost your beauty to the natural aging process, it is just possible that, if you work very hard, you can still *make* yourself desirable, and gain the precious commodity, a man's love." Finally, we are made to feel, it is not we ourselves who will decide whether or not we are beautiful, but someone else. And not only do we hear that voice all around us; we have internalized it. "How can I make myself beautiful so he will love me?" we ask ourselves. It is we women, not the men we know, who ask ourselves anxiously whether we "measure up."

But how could it be otherwise, when the beauty myth on which most women of my generation were raised is one that insists our beauty is determined by others.[3] If few of us literally lost our mothers, as I did, many of my contemporaries had mothers who, no matter how much they may have loved and nurtured their daughters' bodies as small children, taught those daughters, as their bodies became those of women, to know their value (as that of their persons) by their value to others. Susan Brownmiller, in her 1984 book *Femininity*, vividly captures the sense of loss of identity a young woman in our culture may experience with the physical changes in her body which come with adolescence — in this passage, specifically, which come with the development of her breasts:

> Although they are housed on her person, from the moment they begin to show, a female discovers that her breasts are claimed by others. Parents and relatives mark their appearance as a landmark event, schoolmates take notice, girlfriends compare, boys zero in; later a husband, a lover, a baby expect a proprietary share. No other part of the human anatomy has such semipublic, intensely private status, and no other part of the body has such vaguely defined custodial rights. One learns to be selectively generous with breast — this is the girl child's lesson — and through the breast iconography she sees all around her, she comes to understand that breasts belong to everybody, but especially to men. It is they who invent and refine the myths, who discuss breasts publicly, who criticize their failings as they extol their wonders, and who claim to have more need and intimate knowledge of them than a woman herself.[4]

A passage like this one speaks well for the legacy of uneasiness that today's grown feminists of the 1980s and 1990s, women of Brownmiller's generation and my own, are likely to bring to the beauty question. Certainly there is a strong temptation for a feminist today to dismiss the whole issue of "femininity." To care for one's appearance seems to epitomize the definition of woman as a

"sex object" invented and perpetuated by the male-dominated society which has disempowered women for so many centuries. Yet
there is something very sad to me in Brownmiller's portrait of a
young woman who feels that her developing female body is less her
own body because it is celebrated by and shared with others. It
seems particularly sad to think that a woman might feel that because
an infant receives nourishment from her breasts, she herself is
thereby made less whole, that her child has become "the proprietor" of her body. Might not a woman feel an enhanced sense of
herself in the action of nursing — which is not in any way diminished by the passive nature of the activity? And is it not possible to
enjoy being looked at by a man without feeling diminished by his
look? Certainly there are cultures in which the celebration that attends a woman's "coming of age" is a celebration in which she
shares, and which enhances her sense of herself. What Brownmiller's passage about breasts, and other passages like it in contemporary feminist writing speak of — eloquently, if sadly to me — is
a generation of women that has experienced so intensely a threatened usurpation of their bodies — bodies seen as sexual objects, to
be looked at (perhaps to be admired, perhaps to be criticized) but
always judged from without, and even laid claim to physically
"against our will," as the title of Brownmiller's first book about
rape reminds us — that they have felt it necessary to repudiate *any*
claim of their own on their own bodies.

In one respect the feminist movement of the 1960s was adamant
in its defense of a woman's right to a life in the body — eager particularly to insist on women's right to sexual pleasure, in contrast
to the puritanical feminism of an earlier age.[5] A defense of woman's
sexual feeling is, in effect, a defense of her power. Woman's capacity for sexual feeling, those of us who came of age in the early 1960s
discovered, was every bit as strong as a man's: the clitoral orgasm
was the equal to — perhaps even superior to (longer lasting, even
more intense), than the male's ejaculation. But beauty was different;
beauty was suspect. In feminist thinking, from Mary Wollstonecraft in the late eighteenth century, on down to Naomi Wolf in the

late twentieth, beauty has been associated with women's traditional powerlessness. "Taught from their infancy that beauty is woman's sceptre, the mind shapes itself to the body, and, roaming round its gilt cage, only seeks to adorn its prison" (said Wollstonecraft in 1792).[6] Two centuries later Brownmiller echoes the protest against women's traditional concern for appearances: "Appearance, not accomplishment, is the feminine demonstration of desirability and worth. . . . Because she is forced to concentrate on the minutiae of her bodily parts, a woman is never free of self-consciousness. She is never quite satisfied, and never secure, for desperate, unending absorption in the drive for a perfect appearance — call it feminine vanity — is the ultimate restriction on freedom of mind."[7] Naomi Wolf's 1991 book, *The Beauty Myth*, makes the extreme case for the equation between a concern for beauty and woman's powerlessness: in her "Marxist" reading, the male-controlled economic power structure is actually destroying (starving) talented women by selling them the myth that extreme thinness is beauty.

Many contemporary feminist critics write as though all women are like Pecola in that we can only speak about ourselves — and our beauty — through the distorting filter of the dominant (patriarchal) culture.[8] And as with speech, so with seeing: we can only see ourselves, some have argued, through the man's eyes — can only see our bodies through the lens of his "controlling gaze."[9] But, I would argue, women in this country, in this present culture, are not, as a whole, like Pecola. Even in *The Bluest Eye* Morrison gives us the example of another girl-child, the novel's narrator, who though born into the same world, yet is able, if not without difficulty, to discover that "black is beautiful," that *she* is beautiful — as she is. And for the rest of us, for women in the dominant, white culture, if it is not easy for us either to avoid being depersonalized by what has come, in feminine parlance, to be called "the masculine gaze," it is my conviction that we can do it. We can know our own beauty. We can acknowledge that all gazes are *not* alike, that there is a masculine gaze that looks at a woman's body with the eyes of love, as well as one that looks at that body with a desire for mastery over it.[10]

This book might be seen as an effort to prompt a recognition of the difference between the two kinds of gaze, so that, as *feminists*, we can enrich our lives by reclaiming our own beauty.

This book is written out of my belief that appearances not only do but *should* matter. We need not feel guilty, as feminists, if we care about appearances. In fact, beauty matters to me precisely *as a feminist issue*. It matters just because outward beauty is the expression of the inner self, because it is the bearer of identity. I believe it is a very basic need for an adult, as for a child, to be loved *in the body*; and as feminists we are mistaken to deny the validity of that need. I do not imagine that I am asking something easy in asking women, as feminists, to care for appearances. Even if — or perhaps especially if — we have had the strength to throw off the patriarchal vision of women's beauty many of us were schooled in as young women, there is an enormous temptation to throw it *all* away, all concern for appearances. Carolyn G. Heilbrun, a leading American feminist and the general editor of the Columbia Gender and Culture series, in her recent book, *Writing a Woman's Life*, urges us to do just that.[11] She speaks of the relief a woman, who may well have spent the better part of her lifetime "keeping up appearances," feels if she is brave enough in her later years to let go of all that and turn her attention to more important things. "It requires great courage," Heilbrun says, "to ignore one's appearance and reach out, as it were, from behind it to attract and spellbind," for a woman "to dissociate her personhood from her feminine appeal" (p. 54). But I want to insist here at the start of my own study, that to know one's own body merely as a barrier to the "real" self behind it is diminishing and sacrifices an important part of ourselves. The "letting go" Heilbrun speaks of may well be for many of us a necessary first step, but this book is written out of my faith that we can take what may be an even harder second step: we can redefine appearances so we can speak to the world and to those who love us with confidence and affirmation — at any stage of life — *through* our bodies rather than from "behind" them. I would wish for women to resist the impulse to dissociate their personhood from their life in the body; for to do so is to deny (for a man or a woman) our wholeness. Heilbrun expresses her concern in *Writing a Woman's Life* that despite the work of feminist theorists, the majority of American women may not be getting the message — that, though there are precious few available models, it is possible for a woman to pursue in her life the sort of "quest plot" that has always been available to men in our culture. But if women aren't getting the message, perhaps it's because the message we have been receiving from the feminist establishment is not too difficult nor too daunting but, finally, too limiting.

Am I so sure, though, of the rightness of my own message about the value and meaning of appearances? No — or only sometimes: it's what I would *like* to believe, what makes the most sense to me. Can one really be so confident that goodness, or happiness, will blossom into beauty? Is life always that fair? To insist that outward beauty bears an intimate relation to inner spirit is, philosophically, as dubious a proposition as its opposite: that beauty is the gift of fortune, or a god. Even Bembo's interlocutors are quick to point out to him that beautiful women are not always good, ugly ones not always evil. In the present century we need hardly be reminded that some of the most wicked acts of mankind have been committed in the name of the equation between inner virtue and outer beauty. There is, then, and must be, a real uncertainty at the very center of my inquiry. The beauty question is inherently problematic, not because the criteria for beauty are subjective and thus difficult to define, but because the question of beauty's status cannot finally be adjudicated. Since my own interest is in the subjective experience of beauty and not finally in its ontological status, however, all that I can and wish to insist upon here is that if I am to address the beauty question honestly, then the uneasiness and that embarrassment I feel about beauty — which comes from that unresolved, and unresolvable, tension between the objectively perceived state and the subjectively known experience — must itself be *a part* of my subject. And no small part of it. For to maintain an awareness of one's beauty, when that sense is not continually reinforced by the world, *is* difficult; it has certainly been difficult for me. And this book would be false if it did not include the feelings of anger and envy that I and the women writers I will be using as my models in later chapters of this study have felt toward those women who seem simply (unfairly) beautiful, no matter what they might be doing or feeling. I have titled this chapter "The Beauty Myths" to emphasize that I'm not arguing for any one philosophical or aesthetic proposition here. I'm arguing for one way of looking at a particular aspect of life — for one construct, one myth, over another. And it seems essential to include in such a study an exploration of those moments when my own beauty myth seems false to me — to include, that is, the ambivalence, or the essential mystery, about the nature of personal beauty.

Most of the time, these days, I feel happy with the way I look, though finding my way (as it were) back to that original security in the body of the beautiful, loved child has been a difficult and, inevitably, an incomplete journey. There's no such thing as recapturing a lost innocence. I'll never know the security of simply knowing myself as beautiful. In fact, as a small child, I didn't *know* it, didn't think about such things; it was simply there. Even now, when I know that my image of my own body is much more stable, and positive, than in earlier years, I find that my feelings about my body can still fluctuate wildly, with my emotional state.

I suppose that there might be some people who really *are* objectively beautiful all the time. I used to think that my daughter was one of those "simply beautiful" persons — a child with "perfect" features, a glowing complexion, deep blue eyes, long dark lashes, and a kind of inner radiance that made people stop to look at her on the street even when she was a very young child. I used to think then how lucky she was, because she could never know the sort of anxiety about her appearance that I have known. I imagined that a beauty like Ruth's must be immutable — until one day when I went to visit her classroom. She was having a difficult time in her school — we were living in England that year, and everything about the English children and English schooling was alien to her. I walked into the classroom unannounced. She didn't see me, but I saw a plain-featured, dull-looking child sitting on the edge of the group of children gathered round the teacher. And then I knew that *anyone* could be made unbeautiful by unhappiness. Now, as an adolescent, she has a confidence about her appearance I never had at that age. And is that her good fortune? Sometimes I see it in those terms, but I know I'd rather believe it's because she didn't have the sort of painful early childhood that I had. This is to say that I'd like to think it's in part because she had (and has) a mother who loves her and who continues to find her beautiful — not because she is beautiful in the eyes of the world but because she is so fully and increasingly herself.

Beauty as the confirmation of identity: that, for me, is the key. If we can link our sense of being beautiful to our sense of being *most fully* ourselves, rather than with being *denied* our selves, we are in a good position to feel the essential difference between the two kinds of masculine "gaze" to which I referred earlier. Freud's analysis of the psychological root of the aesthetic impulse is, I think, extremely useful here. Our love for beauty, in Freud's view, is a displacement, ultimately, of the infant's auto-eroticism, or the curiosity — and "curiosity" is, I think, the key term here — the infant or young child feels about its own genitals and the pleasurable sensations associated with touching them.[12] As the child grows older and develops object-relations with others, that curiosity is transferred to their genital parts, and especially to the different-looking sexual parts belonging to members of the opposite sex. The love of looking (or "scopophilia") becomes, then, a way in which the child gratifies his or her curiosity; it is tied to the child's growing desire for knowledge of the larger world. And though, in Freud's view, when the child becomes sexually mature, that active pleasure of looking *at* the other comes to dominate in men, while in women scopophilia turns, as it were, back upon itself, so that the passive pleasure in being looked at *by* the other comes to dominate, he recognizes that both sexes retain a capacity for the active pleasure of looking as well as the passive one of being looked at. And both are, for Freud, components of a healthy sexuality. It is only when either pleasure (scopophilia or exhibitionism) becomes the *sole* means by which an individual achieves sexual gratification that an unhealthy situation, or a perversion, develops. Thus while some contemporary feminists have suggested that Freud associates the masculine impulse of scopophilia with "taking other people as objects [and] subjecting them to a *controlling and curious* gaze,"[13] Freud himself never confuses a controlling gaze with a curious one. The two are, in fact, opposites. Which is just where I find his analysis is so useful: it offers us the key with which to distinguish the healthy kind of sexual looking — and of being looked at — from their unhealthy counterparts. Any pleasure that is rooted in a desire for dominion must rightly be termed degrading, both to the one looking and the one looked at. But the love of looking, as Freud describes it, cannot be degrading, as it is rooted not in the desire to control but in curiosity. And curiosity is, quite simply, one of the wonderful, liberating components of the psychic life.

It follows, moreover, that the pleasure we take in *being* looked at, in gratifying another's curiosity about ourselves, is equally affirming, equally liberating. To enjoy being looked at sexually — when the observer looks with a curious rather than a controlling gaze — is to feel the excitement of being discovered, of being known. We have all, I expect, at some time or another, felt the desire to be seen by another as a desire to be worshipped, to be seen as an object of beauty. Such a wish, as it comes ultimately out of a desire for power over another, is simply the corollary to the other person's desire for control over *us* (however it may masquerade itself as homage) and must be recognized as such. It is in such sadomasochistic exchanges of gazing and being gazed at that the issue of women's beauty has been historically enmeshed in Western culture for centuries. But — and this is the burden of my message in this book — it need not be. Not only can we free ourselves from those trammels, we can do much more than that: we can reclaim a wonderful, liberating area of human experience.

Moreover, without arguing for the rightness or wrongness of

Freud's gender differentiation (the eventual predominance of the desire to see in men and the desire to be seen in women), we might notice here an important corollary to that differentiation. Though Freud himself does not draw attention to this fact, the anatomical difference between male and female genitalia reinforces his distinction between the two types of pleasure, active and passive, and gives a special piquancy to the woman's pleasure in being seen. While a gratification of our curiosity about the man's sexual apparatus is easy enough to come by (in a world without clothing, at any rate!), a gratification of that same curiosity about the woman's sexual parts is inherently difficult. A woman's essential sexual organs are hidden — hidden ultimately even from herself: to be seen they must, as it were, wait to be discovered. And though neither he nor she can ever see it all, the man's discovery of the woman's sexual parts (and thus, in Freud's view, of her beauty) can thus be experienced as a symbolic discovery of her (hidden) identity. While to some, the idea that there could be any connection between the discovery of something as complex and unique to the individual woman as her identity could be linked to the discovery of something as "common" as her hidden sexual parts might seem far-fetched or ludicrous, I do think that the feeling, for a woman, of having those hidden parts of herself seen and loved may be very deeply connected to her feeling that she herself is, at the deepest level, known and accepted. In this sense, for a woman, to be looked at and seen as beautiful may feel like a validation of her very self in a way it does not for a man.

To know oneself as beautiful in this second sense is not, as I have already suggested, easy. There are so many obstacles — both from without and from within. And so few models. On the personal level, in order to accomplish it, a woman may need to reach back into her very early past, to before the time she was taught that other, dominant beauty myth from her mother, to remember (if she was lucky enough to receive it) the unconditional love of her body she got as a very small child. For whether we look backward or forward, we all need some image, some model, for this new way of seeing (and loving) our bodies. This book is an attempt to provide such a model by a variety of means. I have looked, first of all, at my own experience with the beauty question at several key points in my life. And, to a lesser extent, I have spoken with women of generations other than my own, at different stages in their lives. Finally, I suppose because I am an inveterate reader of fiction and a literary critic by profession, I have found my most important models for seeing beauty as I wished or needed to find it for myself, not in real life but in the fictions I have read and in the lives of the women who wrote those fictions. In the central sections of this book I discuss the lives and writings of a number of women novelists. They are writers who themselves were searching, in their own struggle with the beauty question, for models. Women novelists, in the late eighteenth and nineteenth centuries, who began writing for a new, female audience did not find in the patriarchal convention available to them any image with which to portray the beauty of their heroines — any more than the present generation of feminists has found an adequate model for beauty in the images produced by "the male gaze" which still pervade our culture. But being women of gifted imaginations, these early novelists invented a new way of describing the beauty of their heroines, or a new convention of heroine-portraiture. And they too had to struggle for it: it was not easy for them, either in their lives or in their writings, any more than it has been for me, to create and hold on to that image of beauty. But it is in the struggle of these early women writers to define the beauty of their heroines (a struggle which reflects issues they were attempting to resolve in their own lives) that I have found the richest confirmation of my own struggle with the beauty question. And, as I hope to demonstrate, their success has much to teach us today — as feminists, as women, as human beings who live in the body and not outside it.

CHAPTER 2

The Woman of Parts

A summer camp for girls I attended at about the age of thirteen had among its end of the season rituals a contest for the perfect — that is, the best-looking — camper. The selection of the perfectly beautiful camper stays in my mind, I think, because it was a very special sort of contest, one which could not be won by any single girl. The winner was a composite creature, endowed with Janey's eyes, Lucy's complexion, and, if memory does not lie, Ellen's mouth. The creation of the ideally beautiful woman out of the assembled parts of a whole group of women is a device with considerable appeal to adolescent girls, who are likely to see their own bodies as a collection of parts which have not yet all come together. And, as the very idea of the composite beauty assumes, they are likely to see their bodies as something separate from themselves. "I have good eyes but bad hair — I really *hate* my hair; if only I had *your* hair: it's so beautiful!"

The privileged adolescent girls I teach talk to one another about their bodies in this way. They compare, evaluate, appraise one another's bodies, part by part, in a way that sounds very familiar to me. And the familiarity of such talk wouldn't be surprising, except that this generation of girls is coming of age well after the explosion of the women's movement in the late 1960s (they weren't even born then!), while my generation grew up before it. Most of these young women have mothers in the workplace, by choice generally rather than by necessity; and my students assume that they will have careers of their own (children too, of course). Much has changed in a single generation for women coming of age. But the "bathroom talk," it would seem, remains pretty much the same. The same girl who argues passionately for Nora's right to a life of self-determination in my classroom discussion of *The Doll House* speaks of her own body as if it were a patient etherized upon a table when she feels she is alone with her friends. In fact, the talk I hear (or over-hear) from today's generation of "liberated" young women about their body parts sounds, if anything, more obsessional and more dissociated than the comparable talk of adolescent girls in my own generation. How disconcerting! I had assumed not only that today's educated, liberated young women would have a more positive image of their bodies than I had at their age, but that they wouldn't "objectify" their body parts as we did — seeing each part as something to be weighed and assessed by an appraising eye, whether their own or that of another. I had assumed that they would be secure in the knowledge of their bodies as an expression of their individual selves. An event which took place a few years ago showed me, though, just how unstable and fraught with ambivalence their sense of their bodies is.

Betty Friedan and Naomi Wolf (as representatives of the old feminism and the new) were invited to our school to speak at a Women's Issues symposium. Naomi Wolf, looking herself not much older than my students and wearing her hair in the same long, loose style, which requires frequent tosses of the head and sweeping gestures of the hand to keep it out of one's eyes, opened the discussion by reading a long excerpt from her then recently published book, *The Beauty Myth*. She read from a section that elaborated her book's central thesis: that the best and the brightest of today's generation of young women (that is, her present audience, my female students) were the victims of a conspiracy on the part of the male-dominated power structure in this country to starve them to death by "selling" them on anorexia, thus creating a famine which, if not quite equal in its dimension to the famines then devastating several third world countries, could be spoken of in the same breath.

I hadn't then read *The Beauty Myth*, but what I heard, coming from the mouth of a self-confessed ex-anorexic, appalled me: Wolf's message seemed to me as wildly exaggerated as it was self-serving. I felt some relief when Friedan, who, for an undeclared reason, refused to assume the podium alongside her younger contemporary but instead talked extemporaneously from her seat among the members of the audience, spoke eloquently of the freedom *she* observed in today's generation of young women about issues involving appearances and sexuality. What she saw was not a generation of young women starving themselves in a competition for men and/or self-extinction but a free-spirited and inventive generation, whose "anything goes" style of dress expressed an infinitely healthier attitude toward appearances than the sweater-set and pearls uniform of her own coming-of-age in the postwar years of the late 1940s and early 1950s. Suggesting that the beauty contest, as she had known it, was dead, Friedan emphasized the need for continued vigilance in combating inequities between men and women in the marketplace.

My women students ignored Friedan. The economic part of her message may — rightly or wrongly — have seemed irrelevant to their own lives. And her observations about this generation's greater freedom of personal style didn't seem to impress them. Their torn blue jeans and long unkempt hair notwithstanding, they knew it was Naomi Wolf's message that spoke to their experience. After the formal discussion was over, the large audience of female students swarmed about Wolf — the first person, they said, to express what they were really feeling. Betty Friedan, doyenne of the women's movement, was left to the company of a few female faculty members, among them myself. The male students in the audience slunk quietly away.

I heard enough of what my students were saying to Wolf that evening to realize that, however distorted her message sounded to my ears, it struck a real chord in theirs and that had to mean something. Some months later, still feeling puzzled and dispirited by what I had seen and heard that evening, I had a long conversation with a former student, who was generous enough to share with me some of her own personal feelings about the beauty question. What she said helped me make sense out of what I had seen at that symposium.

This young woman's mother was a teacher and an ardent feminist. My student spoke of having been taught as a child by both her parents to value her mind, not her physical appearance. Bodies, her parents (and particularly her mother) had taught her, were good for *doing* things. She was, in fact, a superb athlete — a tall, striking looking girl. Her parents had certainly never made her feel that she was an unattractive child; the subject simply hadn't come up. She thought that the values her parents had instilled in her had been basically good ones: she felt confident among her male peers, as ready to speak up in the classroom as to compete on the playing field.

Yet when adolescence came, this student found herself suddenly and surprisingly intensely preoccupied with the issue of her appearance. "When I was with a group of my friends I found myself thinking constantly how pretty *they* were, and that I couldn't possibly compete in that area. If people said how pretty the girls on the team were, I'd say, 'Yes, aren't they' — as if I weren't one of them." She even dismissed her boyfriend's compliments on her appearance: "He just says those things because he's supposed to say them," she assumed. But then she began to wonder whether perhaps she really might be attractive. She began noticing that men looked at her appreciatively when she walked down the street. People even stopped her and asked if she had ever done any modeling. She looked at the pictures of the models with their perfect bodies in the magazine and felt a mixture of incredulity and nausea and a strange rush of pleasure. "They were so perfect; how could I be like that? Could it be that *I* belonged to that category of beautiful people from which I've always excluded myself?" Here was a new discovery about herself, and it gave her a heady kind of pleasure.

This young woman's family had never told her about such pleasure! Significantly, she gave very little thought to whether a particular man might be physically attractive to her: she was much too absorbed by the question of her own desirability. And, as her sense of that desirability had little internal grounding, it could fluctuate wildly, depending on the setting she was in. This was as true (or perhaps even more true) when she was among her female friends than with men. If she were with a group of her girlfriends who in her mind ranked high on the beauty scale, she felt uncomfortably aware of her own low status. On the other hand, if she were in the company of "less desirable" women, her own stock rose proportionally and her sense of self-esteem with it. This was a young woman who, when it came to intellectual assessments of others' merits, could appreciate a wide range of different views. But when the issue was the value of the body, it seemed there was only one yardstick. Different types of physical attractiveness were not interesting or relevant and received little attention in her descriptions of her various women friends. *This* one made it, *that* one didn't; and the crucial but uncertain and therefore intensely anxiety-provoking question was, where did one stand on the evaluative scale?

At about this time, she began to get warnings from her mother, which she resented, about "being taken advantage of" by men. Her mother also criticized her for spending the money that she earned from her summer job on clothes ("How many pairs of shoes do you have anyway?") when she might have been buying books or other more worthwhile things. And the pleasure of experiencing her body as the object of masculine admiration provoked some even more unsettling reactions — in herself. At the time of our conversation she was on summer vacation after her first year in college, and she was feeling as though her life was split into two parts. At college she was her mother's daughter — an outspoken feminist, always on the alert for sexist undercurrents in the comments of fellow male students and quick to censure them. She was discovering, more fully than she had in her high school years, the pleasures of using her good mind. She was loving her courses, particularly those in linguistics and anthropology, where it was interesting to realize how deeply ingrained in our language and culture sexist assumptions are. But this summer, back home and away from the school setting, she had been dating a much older man who, she said, made much of her appearance and treated her "like a doll."

She described to me an interesting sensation she'd had at a party hosted by her new boyfriend, which she thought was typical of herself at this time. He was a man with expensive tastes and expensive friends. She attended the party — a big event — conscious that she was looking her best and that she was getting the sort of attention a very attractive woman gets from men. The problem came when she tried to enter into a "real" conversation with a man. "I felt that if I opened my mouth and said something serious, something I really felt, he wouldn't find me attractive anymore." Interestingly but not surprisingly, she identified "opening her mouth" with being like her mother, and that meant not simply giving away the fact that she *had* a mind, but being the sort of critical person who put other people down. She wanted to think of herself as a more accepting sort of person, but she couldn't find a way to reconcile these different parts of herself. Either she was a disembodied person, speaking as someone with strong convictions of her own and willing to criticize others' views; or she was an attractive woman, enjoying the sensation of being found attractive, and keeping her mouth shut.

I felt I was beginning to understand better what I had seen at the Betty Friedan–Naomi Wolf encounter. Wolf was publicly acknowledging feelings my women students were experiencing themselves, that no one else had acknowledged — feelings they were embarrassed to admit and were confused by but which they knew were very real. The awareness of their bodies as desirable objects, separate from their "real" identity, contradicted everything they'd been taught about the value of appearances by their parents and teachers, as it contradicted their own deeply felt feminist values. (They were feelings that only a very brave young woman could express to her former teacher.) The overwhelmingly gratified response of my women students to Wolf's words was inevitable. My women students do clearly feel trapped in "the beauty myth," as Wolf defines it, and I suspect they experience it *more* intensely than did young women in my generation because they are so much more aware than we were that it *is* a trap. They get such a strong, conflicting message elsewhere — from their mothers (frequently), from such female teachers as myself, and from a highly developed part of their own consciousness. I doubt that these young women (as a group) feel that they are in imminent danger of literally starving themselves in their desire to be the thinnest, most desirable, and least powerful women they can possibly be. I feel confident that the side of them *I* see every day in the classroom is real and not assumed, nor in danger of extinction. But having witnessed the intensity of their response to Wolf and listened carefully to the one student who spoke so frankly to me about her own sense of a divided self, I understand better now the sense of confusion and embarrassment the present generation of "liberated" young women is feeling about the beauty question.

My own reactions to what I see in this new generation of young women are mixed. On the one hand, it seems to me there's nothing intrinsically shameful about the pleasure one takes in having one's body looked at and admired. Shouldn't one be able to enjoy getting back the image of oneself as a beautiful, desirable object in the eyes of another? And why shouldn't a nineteen-year-old girl spend the money she has earned in her summer waitressing job on shoes and jewelry rather than on books or (serious) music? I wonder whether we, as the representatives of the first generation of feminists, have not done our daughters a disservice in teaching them that such pleasures are suspect. Yet then I hesitate. For those feelings *are* often suspect. My student, and all those students who responded so strongly to Wolf's message, did feel that they were betraying their "real selves" by buying into the beauty myth as she defined it. To the extent that they saw themselves as mere objects of another's gaze they saw themselves as depersonalized. And surely something *is* wrong if one feels that as soon as one opens one's mouth and reveals oneself as a person (a thinking, feeling person) the pleasure evaporates. Something *is* wrong if the pleasure in being looked at seems to deny rather than confirm one's sense of one's own individuality.

My own generation of feminists has fought for women's right to be active partners with men in all the varied spheres of life, in the bedroom as well as in the workplace. Perhaps, as a result, we have felt a need to denigrate the passive, narcissistic pleasures women have historically enjoyed—pleasures which seem to us, for good reason, too closely allied to the long history of women's subjugation. Just because the pleasure one receives in being looked at and being seen as beautiful is essentially a passive pleasure, it is easy to confuse the "wrong" kind of gaze with the "right" kind—and therefore all the more crucial that we understand the essential difference between the two. Perhaps in our age a woman needs to know and feel secure in her participation in the pleasures of the active life *before* she can enjoy the pleasures of passive experiences. At the very least, as feminists, I think we have oversimplified the beauty question for ourselves and for our daughters. In later chapters of this book I suggest how we can achieve for ourselves as women, and teach our daughters to enjoy, our own beauty — as the expressions of our own selves. But precisely because we have been trained for so long, as women, to see beauty in its dehumanizing aspect, because that tradition has such a long history in Western culture, I think it is important to look more closely at the history of that dehumanizing "male gaze" — its possible origins and the psychological imperatives which underlie it — before going on to posit a better way of knowing our own beauty, one which confirms rather than denies a curiosity about the self. It is only by understanding more clearly the "wrong" kind of male gaze and the complexity of our responses to it as women that we can begin to appreciate that there *is* another way — a way of enjoying being looked at, and enjoying caring for our own bodies that does not separate us from ourselves.

Because I use women novelists and their fictions as my models for that new way of seeing beauty, I want first to consider the masculine literary tradition against which those women writers were rebelling. For unless one looks closely at the one way of seeing a woman's body, it is very difficult to distinguish it from another, very different way — very different in fact, but, as the confusion of my adolescent students confirms, extremely difficult to disentangle in experience itself. In real life things are rarely clear. The rush of experience — particularly where those feelings least accessible to our rational analysis are involved — overwhelms us; we feel confused. Literature, on the other hand, if we look at it closely, is wonderfully clarifying. I think that by looking closely at the very particular and long-lived literary convention of heroine-portraiture by which men in Western literature have portrayed women's bodies for centuries, we place ourselves in a much better position to understand the psychological imperatives that drive the objectifying "male gaze" at the woman's body, and thus to distinguish it from a very different sort of male gaze, one we need not feel embarrassed to accept. But whatever our choice, it is important to understand what we are choosing, and thus to make our choices freely. By looking closely at the actual mechanism of how a woman's body is objectified in literature, we can help sensitize ourselves to such situations when they occur in real life. For the mechanism is the same.

As I have already suggested, the way to deny a woman her integrity as a person is to see her body as a collection of parts. My "perfect camper" is the heir to a long literary tradition of composite heroines. Western treatises on female beauty often cite the story of the ancient painter Zeuxis, who selected the best features of five different maidens of his native Croton as models for his painting of Helen of Troy.[1] It is to this tradition of the composite beauty Shakespeare teasingly alludes in *As You Like It* when Orlando describes Rosalind as a distillation of "Helen's cheek, but not her heart, / Cleopatra's majesty, / Atalanta's better part, Sad Lucretia's modesty," and concludes: "Thus Rosalind of many parts / By heavenly synod was devis'd, / Of many faces, eyes, and hearts, / To have the touches dearest priz'd" (act 1, scene 2). Unlike Zeuxis and my camp mates, Orlando imagines a single living woman who contains in herself all the best parts; but this perfect woman is still, as he says, a composite creature, made up "of many faces, eyes, and hearts." Throughout Orlando's inventory are continuous reminders that those fabled heroines have their worse as well as their better parts — Helen's cheek is lovely but her heart is hard, Cleopatra has majesty but also pride — suggesting the possibility of imperfection even as they enforce the fact of *his* mistress's exemption from defect. As we thirteen-year-olds understood, the very act of identifying our "perfect" part is a reminder that we have other, less than perfect ones (e.g., "good legs but bad breasts"). This is the language in which the composite beauty (of any age) addresses herself. And it is also the language of the dominant tradition for describing the beautiful heroine in the Western literary tradition.

You might suppose that when a male poet or a novelist wants to describe an ideally beautiful woman he simply imagines the most beautiful woman he can think of, puts his pen to paper, and "describes" her. You might suppose that no particular convention — no shared set of unspoken but highly determining rules or assumptions — is involved here. Or that if anything is conventional about such descriptions, it is features themselves: the blond hair, the blue eyes, and fair skin which we all know are the prerequisites for any heroine worthy of that name in Western literature. But in fact the most powerful conventions are the ones that have to do with the *way* of seeing rather than with *what* is seen. Orlando has not (any more than the judges in my camp contest) actually described any of Rosalind's specific features; yet Rosalind, seeing his verses, recognizes instantly the conventional mode of thinking which controls his versifying — and, being the wise woman that she is, laughs at them. She will eventually teach her lover a better way of looking and of loving.

The significance of a particular style of *seeing*, as opposed to a particular style of *beauty*, is nicely brought out in a comparison of two portraits in which the features of the women themselves are conspicuously different. In fact the "Rebecca-Rowena dilemma" (alluding to the paired heroines of Sir Walter Scott's 1819 novel *Ivanhoe*) has become a kind of catchphrase among literary critics for the predicament of the hero in Western literature who finds himself torn between a blond "angel in the house" and a dark-haired temptress. But if we look at the way Scott introduces us first to the blond Rowena and later to the dark-haired Rebecca in *Ivanhoe*, we may well wonder whether the choice between the two women is not in some sense an illusion of choice. In each case, before we are introduced to the heroine herself, we are prepared to see her through the eyes of the judging man. Rowena is first "seen" in the context of a conversation between two men, a Prior and a Templar: the former is leading his companion (in this novel set in twelfth-century England) to the stronghold of Rotherwood, where the two hope to find hospitality and which is the home of the beautiful Rowena. The preliminary exchange between the two men is saturated with the language of appraisal:

"Of her beauty you shall soon be judge [says the Prior]; and if the purity of her complexion, and the majestic yet soft expression of a mild blue eye, do not chase from your memory the black-tressed girls of Palestine, ay, or the houris of old Mahound's paradise, I am an infidel and no true son of the church."

"Should your boasted beauty," said the Templar, "be weighed in the balance and found wanting, you know our wager?"

"My gold collar," answered the Prior, "against ten butts of Chian wine; they are mine as securely as if they were already in the convent vaults, under the key of old Dennis, the cellarer."

"And I am myself to be judge," said the Templar, "and I am only to be convicted on my own admission that I have seen no maiden so beautiful since Pentecost was a twelvemonth. Ran it not so? Prior, your collar is in danger; I will wear it over my gorget in the lists of Ashby-de-la-Zouche."

"Win it fairly," said the Prior, "and wear it as ye will; I will trust your giving true response, on your word as a knight and as a churchman."[2]

The experience we are being prepared for here is not one of enjoyment, but of evaluation. The question to be asked about the woman is the one my student asked about herself: "What is my value in the beauty contest?" And, as the metaphor of the balance in the *Ivanhoe* passage suggests, the woman's desirability is both objectively determinable and something to be discovered through the action of implied comparison with her competitors — the other women the male viewer has previously assessed. Interestingly, while from the woman's point of view (particularly that of a young woman like my student, or myself in those adolescent years) the judgment may be uncertain or constantly fluctuating, from the man's point of view there is no uncertainty at all. Though the Templar insists on his right to make the final assessment (he will be the judge), the balance metaphor implies an objective standard about which there can be no disagreement. There is an atmosphere of male fraternity here: the Prior trusts the Templar to speak his mind honestly, and thus to win the prize, should he win it, fairly. And subsequently, when Rowena is seen, the Prior underscores the assumption of a masculine consensus: "Said I not so?" he asks the Templar, as the latter, on seeing Rowena enter the dining hall, instantly concedes defeat.[3]

The matching scene which prepares us for our introduction to Rebecca is less elaborate, but again the woman is introduced to us through the eyes of an appraising and a knowing man. "The quick eye of Prince John instantly recognized the Jew, but was much more agreeably attracted by the beautiful daughter of Zion, who, terrified by the tumult, clung close to the arm of her aged father.

"The figure of Rebecca might indeed have compared with the proudest beauties of England, even though it had been judged by as shrewd a connoisseur as Prince John" (chap. 7, p. 93).

Prince John is a "connoisseur" of beauty; we can therefore better trust his judgment. Masculine assessment of the woman is enforced in this instance by the scene's setting — a tournament. The assembled knights agree that whichever man wins in the contest of arms shall be given the right to choose which woman shall win in the contest of beauty and thus occupy "the fair sovereign's throne" (chap. 8).

Though the context in both scenes is obviously sexual, neither of the portrait-painters, the Templar or Prince John, will become romantically attached to the woman he appraises. Nor is either a particularly admirable man. But their estimates are not therefore understood to be partial or in any way defective. The Prior's validation of the viewer's assessment in each case underscores our sense that what each man sees is what any judging man would see. Any man, provided he has sufficient status to participate in the conversation of his peers in the first place, is entitled to pass judgment on a woman. I am reminded of the scene in Delbert Mann's 1955 movie, *Marty*, in which the two men — losers certainly in every sphere including the sexual one — attend a dance and are assigned partners: "I got stuck with a dog," says Angie to Marty. He's a "dog" himself, from a woman's point of view. But in making such a statement Angie asserts his status as a member of the male community and the right thereby conferred on him to evaluate thus conclusively a sexually eligible woman.

In both the *Ivanhoe* scenes, at the moment that the man sees the woman and makes his judgment, the action is suspended; the camera, as it were, "freezes" while the woman is, in effect, forced to "wait" before resuming her own action. And the wait is considerable: in my text Rowena's portrait occupies thirty lines; Rebecca's twenty-five. In the case of Rowena, the sense of the woman being arrested in her movement by the man's appraisal of her is registered explicitly. She enters the banquet hall and is about to take her place; but before she "had time to do so," her progress is interrupted by the portrait followed by the declaration of the Templar's concession of defeat.[4]

While the women thus "stand" waiting, what we get in the formal portraits themselves is in each case a collection of perfectly beautiful parts. Neither Rowena nor Rebecca is actually imagined to have parts borrowed from the bodies of other women: the truly composite beauty is a fantasy creation of schoolgirls and mythmakers. But the *effect* in each case is of a composite ideal, because the unity of the portrait depends in each case not on the fact that each part belongs to this particular woman's body but on the fact that each part is the very *best* part of its kind. Thus "the brilliancy of her eyes, the *superb* arch of her eyebrows, her *well-formed* aquiline nose, her teeth as white as pearl," etc. . . . "— all these constituted a combination of loveliness which *yielded not* to the most beautiful of the maidens who surrounded her" (chap. 7, p. 94, my italics). The adjectives describing the blond Saxon, Rowena, are likewise evaluative rather than descriptive: she is formed in "the *best* proportions of her sex" (not too short, not too tall); her complexion is "*exquisitely* fair" (chap. 4, p. 61, my italics).

That the man's judgment may be negative rather than positive is an important part of his controlling power. Neither Rowena nor Rebecca is a "dog," but they are appraised in a world where the possibility of failure is ever-present. Prince John is a "shrewd connoisseur" of women's figures: we must wonder whether Rebecca will be able to survive such scrutiny. The possibility that Rowena may fail to meet her judge's exacting standards is the first thing we hear about her from the man who will soon do the appraising: "Should your boasted beauty be weighed in the balance and found wanting, you know our wager?" And in Rowena's portrait there are continuing reminders that though she does pass the test, she might not. She is tall, "yet not so much so as to attract observation on account of superior height": a bit taller and she would be too tall. "Her complexion was exquisitely fair, but [fortunately for her!] the noble cast of her head and features prevented the insipidity which sometimes attaches to fair beauties" (chap. 4, p. 61). Negative praise, so unsettling from the point of view of the woman being assessed — and that is just the point! — is reassuring for the assessor, confirming the rightness of his judgments. If the subject of such portraiture is sexual, the setting is that of the law-court rather than the bedroom. We, the readers, are placed in the position of the ultimate judge; the appraising man is her advocate, speaking on behalf of his client but not to her; the woman herself is the silent defendant.

Above all, the sense of reassurance is conveyed by the form of the portraits themselves — that of an orderly catalogue, with each item in its proper place. In each case we move from a general overview of the whole body, to an inventory of parts, as the man's eye travels, step by step, downward. A skeleton outline of Rowena's portrait would read: overview, eye, eyebrow, hair, neck, arms, and then a fade-out at the point at which the body parts meet the covering folds of the dress. Rebecca's portrait follows the same sequence, including a few more details in its downward progression: overview, eye, eyebrow, nose, teeth, hair, neck and bosom, and then again, fade-out. Proper sequencing is a key here. So Leigh Hunt, in his own "Criticism of Female Beauty," will exclaim (with mock facetiousness) that "in attending to the hair and eyes, we have forgotten the eyebrows, and the shape of the head. They shall be despatched before we come to the lips; as the table is cleared before the dessert."[5] The analogy with the Victorian multi-course meal, which is defined by its orderliness as much as by the fact that its ultimate end is to be consumed, is an apt one.

We may better appreciate the psychological function of such an orderly progression by considering the very different effect of a style of heroine portraiture (what we might think of as a sub-convention in the Western literary tradition) in which we see a woman's scattered parts, but in no particular sequence and with no illusion of seeing the whole. In Petrarch's *Rime* we see a glimpse of Laura's beautiful eyes in one poem, her golden hair, white hand or foot in another. When several body parts are mentioned in a single poem, they are not brought into any physical relation to one another. Proust is another of the great chroniclers of love who specializes in the single image or set of selected, unrelated images: the smudge of reddish hair that is Gilberte; something seen passing on the periphery of the narrator's vision, shining black and pale white — Albertine *disparue*. We see only fragments; the woman eludes the man's desire to apprehend her.[6] But in the dominant tradition whose assumptions I am analyzing here, the orderly part-by-part inventory speaks for the success of that mission. She is all there; everything is in its place. The emotional tone of the portrait is one of reassurance, mastery. In Gotthold Lessing's famous eighteenth-century essay on the differing means of achieving verisimilitude in the visual and verbal arts, *The Laocoön*, the author points out that words, unlike pictures, cannot capture a whole image at once; operating as they must through the medium of time, words necessarily "dismember" the image, constrain us to see it piece by piece. Literary artists, as Lessing also recognizes, can find ways, when they wish to do so, of creating the "painterly" effect of a body seen whole.[7] But in the Rowena and Rebecca portraits we might wonder whether dismemberment should be seen not as an unfortunate consequence of the artist's chosen medium but as precisely the desired effect. For "dismembering" describes so well what these portraits in many ways do to their subjects. Which is why women feel, when they are objectified by this sort of masculine gaze, as though they were being dismembered: they are.

From the man's point of view, the goal is not Eros as such, but Eros assimilated into an orderly world where nothing untoward can happen — or Eros made safe. The particular sequence of the progression is important here; it follows the path of the man's sexual advance — though the actual end of his journey is, of course, never reached. As Ariosto, in a franker age, would put it, in the evaluative mode of the convention, "But Argus self might not discern the rest; / Yet by presumption well it might be guessed / That that which was concealèd wàs *the best*" (my italics).[8] Scott's portraits effectively end at the point where the body meets its covering of clothing at the breast. Rowena wears a veil, which can either be wrapped about her face and bosom or, "at the wearer's pleasure," disposed about her shoulders. Rebecca's portrait ends with a more provocative description of her upper garment, whose three upper buttons are left open, "on account of the heat, which something enlarged the prospect to which we allude" (chap. 7, p. 94). On the one hand, there is a teasing play with sexual disclosure in both portraits; on the other hand, though the women may play with mastery, it is clear that the men are really controlling the show. The tone of the Rebecca portrait suggests that the prince is saying, in effect, "I know the game you are up to, but you can't put it over on me." These portraits are less about desire than they are about control. "What if the woman were to open her mouth and say something?" "What if that sexual part which is my destination were to get out of its place, loom too large, perhaps control me?" It can't happen. And thus the *Ivanhoe* portraits are not essentially erotic in feeling. For real eroticism, as Freud reminds us, depends on curiosity, an openness to exploratory impulses, and a willingness to expose oneself to hazard — which is just what such portraits of beautiful women do not do. A few lines from a famous poem by John Donne may point the difference in feeling for us. In the beautiful elegy "To His Mistress Going to Bed" the poet's deliberate mixing up of directional signals —

> *License my roving hands, and let them go*
> *Before, behind, between, above, below.*
> *O my America! my new-found-land . . .*[9]

creates just that sense of discovery which is missing in the *Ivanhoe* portraits — and from the sort of appraisals my students received from men and to which they subject themselves.

In the Rebecca and Rowena portraits each man begins with his curiosity piqued by the possibility of seeing something new and different. The Templar, Brian de Bois Guilbert, has been used to seeing and admiring Eastern beauties. Rowena's style of beauty will not be familiar; she is "more striking perhaps to his imagination because differing widely from those of the Eastern sultanas" (chap. 4, p. 61). Conversely, Prince John has been used to seeing Teutonic beauties, and Rebecca presumably interests him because she too offers the promise of novelty. In the end, however, neither of these men is gratified by novelty but by conformity. The contrast between Rowena and the Eastern beauties is not sustained: she is "formed in the best proportions *of her sex*" (chap. 4, p. 61, my italics). If Rebecca gains Prince John's attention on account of her foreign quality, she holds it because she can compete with or surpass the English beauties on their own terms: her figure "might indeed have compared with the proudest beauties in England" (chap. 7, p. 93). And again: "all these [assets] constituted a combination of loveliness which yielded not to the most beautiful of the maidens who surrounded her" (ibid.). The woman pleases, in the end, not because she surprises the viewer but precisely because she does not surprise him; she conforms to his expectations. She has passed the test, coming in first in each of the prearranged categories.

Consider the striking difference between Scott's initial portraits

of Rowena and Rebecca and the way in which he introduces the
two important male characters in *Ivanhoe*. King Richard and Ivanhoe are both first seen in action and in disguise before we are allowed up close to see their features. When Ivanhoe does disclose
himself at the tournament and is recognized by Rowena, though
the sudden sight of her lover is enough to cause her frame to tremble "with the violence of sudden emotion," Scott does not make use
of this opportunity to survey his hero through a would-be lover's
gaze. What we see is simply "the well-formed yet sun-burnt features of a young man of twenty-five . . . amidst a profusion of
short fair hair" (chap. 12, p. 146). In the female portraits the question at issue is: "Is this woman the best, the fairest lady of them all?"
And the question is in each case resolved by the looking, the visual
appraisal, itself. But in the male portraits the question is, "Who or
what sort of a man is this?" King Richard, as the black knight, takes
off his helmet, to reveal to his interlocutor features and a form
which express "altogether the look of a bold, daring, and enter-
prising man" (chap. 16, p. 175): appearances are important not in
themselves, but as clues to character.

Scott introduces his heroines in the particular way that he does
because he is participating in a convention for heroine-portraiture
which has a long history in Western literature. To know the origins
of that convention (as of any convention) is to understand better its
meaning, the assumptions which underlie it. Some have traced the
origins of the sort of heroine-portraiture we see in *Ivanhoe* to the
poetry of late antiquity. But while several of the features of the heroine (the golden hair, the milk-white skin, the broad forehead and
bright eye) are indeed present in such poems as the elegy for his
mistress by the sixth-century poet Maximian,[10] the features of the
portraits themselves (particularly, the catalogue style which "fixes"
as it inventories the woman's parts) are not.[11] Others have found a
source for the later catalogues in Hebraic poetry, particularly in
the catalogue of the bride in *The Song of Songs*.[12] Here we do find
the catalogue form. But to recall just a few of the items in the bib-

lical inventory of the bride's beauties is to feel their difference from
the effect of part-by-part inventory in the Rowena and Rebecca
portraits:

> Your hair is like a flock of goats
>   moving down the slopes of Gilead.   (*RSV* 4:1)

> Your neck is like the tower of David,
>   built for an arsenal,
> whereon hang a thousand bucklers,
>   all of them shields of warriors.   (4:4)

> Your two breasts are like two fawns,
>   twins of a gazelle,
>   that feed among the lilies.   (4:5)

To read these biblical verses is to realize that a catalogue of parts
need not feel disempowering. The serial similes in *The Song of
Songs* have the effect of enlarging and energizing the image of the
woman rather than diminishing her. She is associated with the fertility of nature and the military might of Judea. What such a comparison does force us to realize is that, in the portrait of the beautiful
woman which dominates the later Western tradition, the idea of
woman's beauty as an expression of her fertility plays no part. She
does not possess that feminine power any more than other kinds of
power. She is the helpless (infantile) virgin.

The real source for our convention is neither in Hebraic nor in
classical texts but in Christian ones, specifically in the French romances of the twelfth century. This is a period from which we date
the decline of the feudal system and the beginnings of what we still
mean when we speak today of "Western culture." It is a period in
which sexual love is rediscovered as a possible literary topic and assimilated to the Christian ethos. And it is also a period in which the
woman's body is viewed by the man, as in neither the Hebraic nor
classical worlds, as something powerfully attractive but also dangerous, the source at once of his salvation and his damnation, his
pleasure and his pain. In other words, this is just the sort of world

in which a man's strongest impulse might well be to familiarize rather than to celebrate the woman's body, to assert some control over an area of his experience where control cannot be taken for granted.

Here we may take as a model not a portrait from one of the romances themselves, but a recipe for such portraits by an English rhetorician, Geoffrey of Vinsauf. It is Geoffrey, writing in the early thirteenth century, who articulates in his *Poetria Nova* the central precept of the portrait as an inventory of perfectly beautiful parts, arranged in descending order.[13] Geoffrey's ideally beautiful woman, like Rowena and Rebecca, is, in W. S. Gilbert's nice phrase, "everything she ought to be and nothing that she oughtn't-oh!" Her proportions are the *best* proportions. If we ask how large her waist is, the answer is not given in inches: it is "so slim that a hand may encircle it," which (even allowing for hyperbole) implies masculine guardianship. Any possibility of excess, of possible deviation from the ideal, is warned against. Praise is couched in negative terms: her nose should be "not too long nor too short," her lips rounded but not *too* rounded; her shoulders, "conforming to beauty's law," should not "slope in unlovely descent, nor jut out with an awkward rise." In sum, says Geoffrey, "Let the radiant description descend from the top of her head to her toe."

But, of course, it is not *all* surveyed: it almost never is.[14] As Geoffrey descends past the region of the waist, he comments: "For the other parts I am silent — here the mind's speech is more apt than the tongue's." In his very discretion we may note, however, that the portraitist assumes the proprietor's role. These parts seem less hers — to give or to withhold through her actions, as his — to give or withhold through his speech. And having passed that critical zone, the lower parts of her body receive perfunctory treatment: "let her leg be of graceful length and her wonderfully tiny foot dance with joy at its smallness."

In the witty and outrageous poem "Loves Progress" (c. 1610), John Donne proposes that instead of traveling downward, the poet reverse his progress and begin at the bottom rather than the top.

The advantage, Donne points out, is speed. Though you may travel farther by taking "this empty and Ætherial way," Donne advises the poet, you will not be retarded either by the delaying strategies or by the secondary attractions located in the upper regions.[15] In effect, Donne is saying to the poets of the traditional convention: "You don't really want what you pretend to want, or you wouldn't go about it in that leisurely, methodical way." "Loves Progress," on the other hand, is a poem about rape; the conventional poets who follow the downward journey and perforce must deal with those upper regions (whatever they really want) are at least dealing in the coin of seduction. Alice Colby, who has made an exhaustive study of the twelfth-century French romances, notes that the one romancer who does actually say something about the woman's genitalia uses a diminutive form to describe that region ("petitet").[16] "What shall I say, asks Hué de Rotélande, of that part beneath which is called the 'cunet'? That I think it was a pretty little thing"[17] — thus nicely assimilating this part to the world of the small and the safe.

If the beautiful woman is one whose sexuality poses no threat, it is not surprising that her antitype should be drawn in opposite terms. From another, slightly earlier French rhetorician, Matthew of Vendôme, comes a recipe for the supremely ugly woman.[18] As we move, once again, systematically downward, we descend from a hairless head to the rough forest of the eyebrows, past ears flowing with filth, rheumy eyes, flat nose, wrinkled cheeks, drooping lips, decayed teeth, mangy neck, and two "matching bladders, counterfeit breasts." But having passed those zones, the observer does not in this instance avert his gaze discreetly from the sexual parts. And while up to this point Ugliness personified has been presented as a figure of decrepitude, a distasteful but presumably harmless old woman, what we see in that place is fully alive, premenopausal if not fecund — and menacing: "Her belly looms with lust. . . . Her hollow trap gapes with numberless hairs, / The flow of sulfurous whirlpool is red. / The descent to the flank bristles with briars; / Cerberus howls; the gaping hollow spouts forth dregs." And then, after that vision of terror, we return to the image of decrepitude, and get the usual perfunctory treatment of the lower extremities — just a glimpse of a stiffened knee joint and the digits of hands and feet gnarled by gout. The all-consuming lust, which is at the real center of this portrait of female ugliness, is in the best medieval antifeminist tradition, and I do not quote Matthew's version of it to expose this caricature once again, but to suggest how such a vision of the ugly woman elucidates our vision of her companion, whose description immediately precedes hers. More than that, I think we may go so far as to say that it is the wild, threatening sexuality of this ugly woman which "begets" her opposite. If the ugly woman does not often, as here, stand literally behind her beautiful companion, her shadow does nevertheless stand behind the beautiful woman everywhere in the patriarchal convention, as in the imaginations of the men who conceive her.

Is it a coincidence that one of the few portraits in the Western literary tradition of an ideally beautiful body that does convey an erotic sense of contact between the gazer and the object of the gaze is of a man's body, not of a woman's? In Christopher Marlowe's portrait of Leander (1598), the visual apprehension of each part is absorbed into a fuller sensory engagement with the body, including the sense of taste and particularly that of touch, so we are led, as we read, to the very threshold of lovemaking itself:

> His body was as straight as Circe's wand;
> Jove might have sipped out nectar from his hand.
> Even as delicious meat is to the taste,
> So was his neck in touching, and surpassed
> The white of Pelops' shoulder. I could tell ye
> How smooth his breast was, and how white his belly,
> And whose immortal fingers did imprint
> The heavenly path with many a curious dint
> That runs along his back . . .[19]

In these last lines Leander's vertebrae are not so much seen as, through the recollection of the action involved in their original creation, caressed. Again we see evidence that a part-by-part inventory does not *have* to be static, distancing. Here it is hard not to suspect that Marlowe's own homosexuality is part of what allows him to portray his hero's body in *Hero and Leander* (as he does not his heroine's) so freely, in such erotic terms. Of course homosexual love is not by definition immune from those same anxieties about possession and being possessed that create the distancing, or objectifying, in the portraits of women we have been analyzing in this chapter. But one might wonder whether in our culture it is not, at the least, *harder* to dismember men's bodies in the way that women's bodies have been — and continue to be — dismembered.

If one wants to "feminize," or disempower, a man's body, the thing can be done much more subtly and profoundly than by dressing him up in the clothing of the opposite sex. In *Joseph Andrews* (1742) Fielding makes the passion of the fifty-year-old Lady Booby for her seeming-servant appear all the more ludicrous by detailing the latter's charms in the language of conventional heroine-portraiture, beginning with the over-all, nonsensical image of a youth "of the highest degree of middle stature," and then detailing his parts in descending order, from hair "displayed in wanton ringlets down his back," to a "high forehead," a Roman eye, "teeth white and even," lips "full, red and soft," and a "beard only rough on his chin and upper lip."[20] It is not Joseph's fair hair and white teeth that declare his effeminacy: it is the way the features are arranged.

Right up until the Industrial Revolution, in the romances and in the novels which follow them, the physical features of heroes and heroines are much more striking for their similarities than for the differences between them. The white unblemished skin, the clear eyes, even the teeth (present rather than absent!) praised in heroes and heroines alike attest to a life of privilege, exemption from the hard, back-breaking labor, and the scourge of disease that marked the masses of those who labored on the land. In these early portraits it is the form that announces sexual differentiation, not the features themselves. The rhetoricians (and the poets) are aware of the danger of doing to a man's body what they do, as a matter of course, to a woman's. Matthew tells us that "the giving of approval to the form of the feminine sex ought to be amplified . . . it ought to be restrained in the masculine sex" (p. 67). To dismember a body is to disempower it; and while this may be just what a male poet wants to do with his heroine's body, it is not (presumably) what he wants to do to his hero's.[21] The dangers — or the peculiar advantage, depending on one's purposes — of doing to a man's body what is done as a matter of course to a woman's is something writers have long known how to exploit. In Chaucer's fourteenth-century *Romance of the Rose*, a poem heavily indebted to earlier French romances, Idleness and other female guardians of felicity receive extended "top-to-toe" portraits, while Mirth, a beardless youth who occupies an adjacent post, is deliberately feminized by a similar portrayal.[22]

What changes in the postindustrial age is that the features inventoried in these early portraits become markers for a sex rather than a class associated with the exemption from work.[23] But here a crucial difference must be registered. When the signs of leisure become the defining features of a group whose leisure is enforced, tokens of power become tokens of powerlessness. The beautiful woman admired in the postindustrial age for her fair, unblemished skin is a prisoner in her leisurely world.

In the course of the nineteenth century, "beauty" becomes a term increasingly relegated to the woman alone, while "handsome," which up through the eighteenth century defines a particular style of beauty which might be found in either sex, a beauty with associations of grandeur, now gets drawn into service as the term for an exclusively masculine ideal of good looks.[24] (The popular phrase of the 1960s, "beautiful people," is exceptional in the modern period in that it designates men as well as women, and is an interesting reversion to the earlier usage: "beautiful people" are upper-class men and women of leisure.) Each term in the postindustrial triad for the ideally attractive man — "tall, dark, and handsome" — marks differentiation along sexual rather than social lines: he is tall rather than short (as women are meant to be); dark rather than blond (as women are meant to be); "handsome" rather than "beautiful" (as women are meant to be). And perhaps both sexes have been the losers for such an evolution — as manly good looks are defined in such a way as to rule out an earlier acceptance of the pleasures of decorating the body, and womanly good looks are defined in such a way as to rule out action in the world.

But sex roles in our society, despite all the resistance, are changing. It would be easy to downplay the fashion in modern advertising and in real life for a more athletic-looking body in women, to see it as just another look, perhaps even another "cop-out," a betrayal of true liberation. But when I look at my present generation of women students, I certainly see a style of beauty that defines itself in more active, physical terms. To me this suggests that, however conflicted they may be about their appearances, these young women are defining their bodies — *and therefore themselves* — in more active, assertive terms. The student whose feelings about her body I spoke of at the start of this chapter is a good example. Surely one reason others stop to look at her on the street has to do with her striking carriage: she carries her height and long limbs with the pride and grace of the athlete she is. If those limbs are free of fat, they have plenty of muscle on them. Everything about her is in motion, including the long, loose swinging hair that is such an emblem of this generation. It speaks to me at once of sensuality and of freedom. I suspect that as this young woman grows a bit older, she will come to realize that her beauty of mind and of body are really in harmony with one another. Even now, I suspect that to a greater extent than she can yet see, she is attractive to men just because of the way her body, like her mind, radiates energy. I think, by contrast, of a female colleague, somewhat older than myself, who told me of the embarrassment she had felt as a young woman, when traveling on her own in Israel in the 1930s, and thumbing a ride from a convoy of soldiers, at having to be lifted onto their truck, like a little child. And I certainly know that in my own life the fashion for women's fitness couldn't have come at a better time. I was in my late twenties, feeling betrayed by my body for its failure to produce the child I wanted so badly. I started swimming laps, and found that I loved it. I also found myself, for the first time in my life, part of a group of women who were all naked together — dressing and undressing, showering, using the sauna. I know that this experience didn't make the pain of not being able to conceive a child go away. But looking back, I realize that this period marked the beginning of a new feeling of pride in my body and in what I could do with it, and (perhaps equally important) a new sense of feeling at home in my body in a comfortable setting with other women. These are feelings which have stayed with me, and — at least as much as my sexual experiences with men — are linked to whatever sense I have now of knowing (or re-knowing) my body as a beautiful body.

In concluding this chapter, I want to suggest just how enduring is the particular style of heroine-portraiture we see in the Rowena and Rebecca passages in the Western patriarchal literary tradition. If we can trace its origins back to the medieval romances of the twelfth century,[25] this convention flourishes luxuriantly in Renaissance epic and lyric poetry,[26] from whence it descends to the novel, where it survives in such male masters of the genre as Fielding in the eighteenth century[27] and Thackeray in the nineteenth.[28] I cannot be the only female reader of *Tristram Shandy* (1760–67) who picked up my pencil and drew my own picture of the Widow Wadman on the famous blank page where Stern invites his "gentle[man] reader" to " — call for pen and ink — here's paper ready to your hand. — Sit down, Sir, paint her to your own mind — as like your mistress as you can — as unlike your wife as your conscience will let you — 'tis all one to me — please put your own fancy in it."[29] But, in so doing, I knew I was breaking the rules! Stern's invitation, couched in the confidential terms of conversation between one man and another, is less open-ended than the narrator suggests, since these terms already prescribe the lineaments of the image that can be drawn on this *tabula rasa*.

Two portraits from our own century may serve to remind us how very much alive this patriarchal convention of heroine-portraiture still is. The first is the famous passage from James Joyce's *Portrait of the Artist* (1916), where Stephen Daedalus sees an unknown girl on the beach. In one respect this portrait is not typical of patriarchal heroine-portraiture: the evaluative modifiers are absent here. This girl is not, for the observer, the same as all the others only more so. What Stephen sees is something unique: in Joycean terms, an epiphany. But the central core of the convention's way of seeing things is present: the inventory of body parts serves to make the experience of sexuality into something that feels safe and reassuring (however profoundly moving) for the man.

A girl stood before him in midstream, alone and still, gazing out to sea. She seemed like one whom magic had changed into the likeness of a strange and beautiful seabird. Her long slender bare legs were as delicate as a crane's and pure save where an emerald trail of seaweed had fashioned itself as a sign upon the flesh. Her thighs, fuller and softhued as ivory, were bared almost to the hips where the white fringes of her drawers were like featherings of soft white down. Her slateblue skirts were kilted boldly about her waist and dovetailed behind her. Her bosom was as a bird's soft and slight, slight and soft as the breast of some darkplumaged dove. But her long fair hair was girlish: and girlish, and touched with the wonder of mortal beauty, her face.

She was alone and still, gazing out to sea; and when she felt his presence and the worship of his eyes her eyes turned to him in quiet suffrance of his gaze, without shame or wantonness. Long, long she suffered his gaze and then quietly withdrew her eyes from his and bent them towards the stream, gently stirring the water with her foot hither and thither. The first faint noise of gently moving

water broke the silence, low and faint and whispering, faint as the
bells of sleep; hither and thither, hither and thither: and a faint flame
trembled on her cheek.

— Heavenly God! cried Stephen's soul, in an outburst of profane
joy. — [30]

Each man appropriates the woman for his own purposes, and
Stephen's are at least as much literary as they are sexual. But the
girl's sufferance of his gaze, in which shame and wantonness are introduced as possible responses to be exorcised, confirms what
every line of the passage declares: she has no choice but to suffer it.
Stephen perceives her parts in top-to-toe sequence, inverse order.
The girl's skirts are "boldly" gathered up, as if to expose parts generally hidden. But what Argus with his hundred eyes sees is all softness and slightness, the realm of the diminutive, of the pure and the
safe. The images of emerald and ivory have their place in the private
iconography of Joyce's *Portrait*, but also in the world of the patriarchal convention, where they have associations of treasures to be
held, hoarded, inventoried. Such a vision of woman is certainly relevant to a protagonist whose fantasies — and actual experiences —
of women have hitherto been in the unsettling world of prostitutes.
Stephen's vision of the woman on the beach comes to him as something wonderfully surprising, but it is also profoundly reassuring.
No claim at all is made here that the nameless woman on the beach
has an independent life of her own; we read her entirely through his
perspective, as the answer to his needs.

And, from a novel even closer to our time, Nabokov's *Lolita*
(1955) — an appropriation of the woman's body by the observing
man with a vengeance! It is the moment in which Humbert Humbert first sees his darling's mother and his eventual bride, Charlotte
Haze. She is written off in that first glance. And Nabokov does it,
brilliantly, by introducing the lady in the act of descending the
stairs. The narrator's eye, traveling upward and cataloguing her
parts in sequence, as they appear to him in reverse order once again,
does only more graphically what such seeing always does to the
woman: it effectively cancels any possibility of independent mo-

tion, or progress, on her part: ". . . there came from the upper landing the contralto voice of Mrs. Haze, who leaning over the banisters inquired melodiously, 'Is that Monsieur Humbert?' . . . Presently, the lady herself—sandals, maroon slacks, yellow silk blouse, squarish face, in that order—came down the steps, her index finger still tapping upon her cigarette."[1] H.H. follows this up with "I think I had better describe her right away, to get it over with." The preparation for his eventual murder of Charlotte, another act to be "got over with" is anticipated in this initial portrait.

I want to conclude my own inventory of portraits with what is, for me, the most extraordinary, in some sense the most moving in the gallery. Like many portraits in the convention, this one gives us a strong sense of the powerlessness of the woman being apprehended by her male portraitist. But here the effect is terrifying because this time it is something we are *meant* to feel and protest against. A man is constructing the portrait, as customarily, in the presence of another man. But we are not invited into their circle. Our sympathies now are with the woman, whose voice we have heard elsewhere in the novel—whose novel, in fact, this really is. The book is Samuel Richardson's *Clarissa* (1747–48), and the portrait occurs in a letter, from Clarissa's rakish admirer and eventual seducer, Lovelace, to his confidant, Belford. Here particularly we feel the atmosphere of the law court invading what pretends to be a scene of haut-bourgeois domesticity, with the lover as advocate, the friend to whom he writes as judge ("thou shalt judge"), and the woman as silent defendant. But in *Clarissa* the situation is complicated by the fact that we can't simply listen along with Belford, judging with him; we can't feel comfortable in the role the convention assigns to us, or here we might say, forces us into.

Lovelace establishes his credentials at the start by assuming proprietorship of Clarissa's body and placing her on the evaluative ladder; she is just one (if the best) of many women he has criticized, taught to dress and undress. The roles of portraitist and seducer merge here, as the man who clothes and unclothes the woman assumes the right to "dress" her (and undress her) in his sketch:

"Thou shalt judge of her dress as, at the moment I first beheld her, she appeared to me, and as, upon a nearer observation, she really was. I am a critic, thou knowest, in women's dresses. Many a one have I taught to dress, and helped to undress. Expect therefore a faint sketch of her admirable person with her dress.'"[2] Then begins the portrait proper, and Lovelace proceeds in the typical evaluative mode of the convention, certifying not only Clarissa's illustrious beauty but her illustrious, model health:

> Her wax-like flesh (for, after all, flesh and blood I think she is), by its delicacy and firmness, answers for the soundness of her health. Thou hast often heard me launch out in praise of her complexion. I never in my life beheld a skin so *illustriously* fair. The lily and the driven snow it is nonsense to talk of: her lawn and her laces one might indeed compare to those: but what a whited wall would a woman appear to be who had a complexion which would justify such unnatural comparisons? But this lady is all glowing, all charming flesh and blood; yet so clear that every meandering vein is to be seen in all the lovely parts of her which custom permits to be visible.   *(pp. 221–22)*

There is something peculiarly unsettling here, as Lovelace in the idiom of the convention assumes possession over the physical attribute we would most think of as belonging to Clarissa herself (as to my student): the healthy glow which is the sign of her inner vitality. Lovelace goes beyond the usual assumption of proprietorship in the convention, established by seeing the woman as a collection of parts. Between the lines of the static portrait we see the signs of a struggle for possession of a woman's spirit, which becomes more palpable as the portrait continues. Having detailed her hair and head-dress, gown and earrings, the handkerchief (made by Clarissa's own hands) which covers her shoulders and breasts, Lovelace makes the usual allusion to the beauties unseen but presumed best: ". . . a white handkerchief, wrought by the same inimitable fingers, concealed—O Belford! what still more inimitable beauties did it not conceal! And I saw, all the way we rode, the bounding heart (by its throbbing motions I saw it!) beneath the charming umbrage" (p. 222). While Lovelace alludes to those "still more inimitable beauties concealed" by Clarissa's covering handkerchief, what he actually sees, without quite acknowledging it as such, is the seat not of sexuality (the woman's breasts standing in, as in the Rowena and Rebecca portraits, for her sexual parts generally) but of feeling — more precisely, of fear. And we may notice that the setting has shifted, without any acknowledgment but most significantly, from the earlier period of Lovelace's first acquaintance with Clarissa, a setting in which a formal portrait may be made ("at the moment I first beheld her") to the present time, where we see Clarissa in the act of being abducted, "as we rode," in Lovelace's coach. It is happening *now*, and the idea of capture, already implicit in the formal portrait, takes on new urgency. Then, finally, having dispatched coat, shoes, "the prettiest foot in the world," and charming arms in a pair of black velvet muffs, Lovelace concludes the portrait with her hands — left bare: "Her hands, velvet of themselves, thus uncovered the freer to be grasped by those of her adorer" (p. 222). It is the perfect ending: the hands left free — "free" to be grasped by his. And it leaves us with a powerful sense of Clarissa's own struggle to free herself, a struggle which, as this passage implies, is doomed to failure. What is remarkable, though, about this portrait is that we do see that struggle; we see what is happening, and feel the horror of it, from the woman's point of view — which now is also the author's point of view — even in the man's portrait where she remains as silent as any woman who sits passively for her portrait in the patriarchal convention.

In this sense, Richardson may be said to use the convention to redirect its purposes. Lovelace makes Clarissa safe for himself; but we want her freed — and his exploitation of the convention's traditional resources only intensifies that desire. To know what Clarissa is feeling here we have to read between the lines. Richardson's effect is particularly powerful just because he does not give her her own voice in this passage. The text becomes, in effect, the bars of the woman's prison-house. To hear the woman's own voice directly, to know her feelings about being looked at, about being or not being beautiful, we have to go outside the patriarchal convention, to a new convention of heroine-portraiture developed by women writers.

CHAPTER 3

Beauty and Identity:
The Woman's Perspective

*W*omen novelists in the mid-eighteenth century, addressing a new audience of educated women readers, found themselves, like Shakespeare's Rosalind in the woods of Arden, surrounded by portraits, or sonnets carved on trees, ill-shaped to serve their needs. They knew what it meant — and how it would feel — for Rosalind to see an image of herself "of many parts devis'd . . . to have the touches dearest priz'd." And if some women novelists were content to perpetuate in their own fictions the patriarchal convention of heroine-portraiture (for women, we know, have often internalized the disempowering masculine inventory of their own body parts),[1] increasingly, as time went on, others — particularly the greatest, most creative women novelists — were not. The ultimate destiny of their heroines might still be the perfect marriage, but that perfect marriage was itself defined in new terms. These were heroines who could think and act for themselves; they were centers of consciousness in their own worlds, not rewards for a hero's good performance.[2] The woman novelist, who has lived a woman's life, has lived not only a different social, emotional, and mental life: she has lived a different life in the body. In the simplest terms, she has known her body from the inside out, rather than the outside in. She may, at times, see her body from the outside, as a collection of parts; but she does not in fact experience it that way. Whether she feels herself to be beautiful or ugly — and such feelings will, most likely, be an important part of her subjective life — she will experience both her beauty and her ugliness from a very different perspective than that of an observing man. And sooner or later, she will want, in her fiction, to find a way of portraying that different life in the body — a vital part of her own experience. If she is a great novelist, she will give us a sense of the feel and texture of her own subjective life in the body such that she will make us think we live there too. Surveying the uncharted terrain waiting to be explored by the woman novelist of the future, Virginia Woolf, in her 1929 essay *A Room of One's Own*, says,

> Above all, you must illumine your own soul with its profundities and its shallows, and its vanities and its generosities, and say what your beauty means to you or your plainness, and what is your relation to the ever-changing and turning world of gloves and shoes and stuffs swaying up and down among the faint scents that come through chemists' bottles down arcades of dress material over a floor of pseudo-marble. For in imagination I had gone into a shop; it was laid with black and white paving; it was hung, astonishingly beautifully, with coloured ribbons. Mary Carmichael [the name Woolf assigns her imaginary future woman novelist] might well have a look at that in passing, I thought, for it is a sight that would lend itself to the pen as fittingly as any snowy peak or rocky gorge in the Andes.[3]

Woolf saw such a fictional rendering of a woman's subjective experience as the challenge for a new generation of women novelists. But the writers Woolf addresses — the serious women writers of the later twentieth century, those whose fictions I turn to for images of women's lives today — Doris Lessing, Nadine Gordimer, Cynthia Ozick, to name a few — spend little time in dress shops, devote little space in their fictions to telling us what a woman's beauty may mean to her, or her ugliness. Those traditional elements of women's subjective experience are just the ones they are most likely to avoid. And I, for one, miss seeing in the fiction of my contemporaries the sort of feminine experience Woolf describes here presented in anything but critical terms. My daughter and I will never enter a shop remotely resembling the one Woolf describes, but we do have a lot of fun browsing through the pictures in the latest J. Crew catalogue, purchasing perhaps a beautiful bathing suit or T-shirt rather than gloves or ribbons. The play of a given color or texture of fabric against the skin tone and texture of one's own body is a part of my life experience as a woman I have no wish to repudiate. Unlike some feminists, I do not look forward to the day, either in my own personal life or in the life of my sex as a whole, when we can stop caring about such things. We have so much of the taking off of women's clothing in contemporary fiction, so little of its putting on! Yet the latter seems to me an equally compelling subject, far from trivial, and rich in the emotional weight it can carry — a subject, in other words, good for fiction. The beauty question is, I suspect, not only for myself but for most of us, not so much one of "what our beauty *or* our plainness means to us," but a question of what our beauty *and* our plainness mean to us — a more complex and therefore even more interesting area of emotional experience than Woolf's notation suggests.

Unlike Woolf, I have found myself looking backward rather than forward for attention paid to the beauty question in women's fiction. Though the women writers of the late eighteenth and nineteenth centuries have little to say about the subjective experience of women's life after marriage, and do not address women's sexual feelings in explicit terms, they are a lot more frank than writers of our own generation in dealing with the beauty question. Jane Eyre doesn't think it is odd that she should care about her appearance, and shares with the reader very openly her complex feelings about her "plainness." Beauty is not the embarrassment to an earlier generation of feminists that it is to the present one. They may well feel that society places too high a value on women's beauty; but they are, I think, less likely than we to confuse men's visions of women's bodies with women's own feelings about their bodies.

One might ask whether this talk about beauty in women's fiction of those earlier centuries is simply the novelists' vehicle for talking about the taboo subject of sex. As Freud's analysis reminds us, there is an area of overlap between the two areas of experience. Yet the farther we travel toward sexual consummation, the farther

we travel from the personal and social worlds in which much of our
lives are lived. That impersonality (or going beyond the realm of
the personal, as D. H. Lawrence would have it) is part of the wonder and essential mystery of sex. But when the lights go out, we
leave behind us all those feelings about how we look and feel about
our bodies in the daylight, in the mirror's reflection, when our
clothes are on, or when we're *in* the world rather than sheltered
from it. We leave behind the comparison of our bodies to others'
bodies — a relief, perhaps, but still a loss of something that's an important part of our daily experience. And we leave behind us the
question of beauty's fairness or unfairness: she may have a beautiful
face, or not; it doesn't matter anymore. For beauty might be described as the special terrain where sexual and social and personal
issues all converge. And if we think of the experiences which confirm our sense of being at home in our bodies, feeling the inner and
outer parts of our selves in harmony with one another, I think those
experiences are at least as likely to occur outside the bed as inside it.

Some fifty years before Charlotte Brontë insisted that "it was
wrong, *even morally wrong*," for a novelist to make a heroine beautiful "as a matter of course," Fanny Burney, a major influence on
later women novelists and a popular writer as well as an important
one in her own right, struggled with the question of beauty's "fairness" in her third novel, *Camilla* (published in 1796). "The unfortunate Eugenia" is not the heroine of Burney's novel: for the plain
woman to assume the center of the fictional stage we must wait for
Jane Eyre. On the other hand, while Jane may be defiantly "plain,"
Burney has given Eugenia (as Dickens would give Esther Summerson a century later) one of the most dreaded, disfiguring dis-
eases of the age: smallpox. If not the heroine, Eugenia is also not a
minor figure in this novel: she is the heroine's youngest sister. The
numerous twists and turns of her progress, as she moves toward
her own destination of a happy marriage, take up almost as much
space — and constitute as interesting a story — as Camilla's own
wayward course along the same path.

Eugenia is — or rather, becomes — an ugly woman; ugliness is thrust upon her: for Burney goes out of her way to enforce the lesson that it is *not the woman's fault.* The onset of Eugenia's affliction is the subject of the novel's opening chapter. The three Tyrold sisters and their brother, the children of a good but modestly situated clergyman living in the country, are celebrating the tenth birthday of the eldest daughter, Camilla, with festivities held at the large estate of their father's bachelor brother, Sir Hugh. As the elder brother, Sir Hugh is the heir to the large Tyrold fortune and has declared the young Camilla his heir. As a special treat, the well-meaning but foolish uncle takes the children for an outing in his coach, in the course of which they stop at a fair in the suburbs. Here he goes against the express instructions of their mother, who has had her elder children inoculated against the smallpox, but has ordered that Eugenia, being still too young and of too delicate a constitution for that protective measure, be "scrupulously kept . . . from all miscellaneous intercourse in the neighborhood."[4] Sir Hugh, however, an indulgent man of the old school, pooh-poohs the sensible mother's precaution, thus revealing his benighted attitude toward the new and still highly controversial practice of inoculation. She "will be sure to have it when her time comes, whether she is moped up [inoculated] or no," he blandly asserts. "And how did people do before these new modes of making themselves sick of their own accord?" Burney's novel is a plea for a modern, rational approach to child rearing — as it is for a rational approach to the beauty question. The little Eugenia is permitted to leave the shelter of her uncle's coach; her innocent voice is shortly heard calling out to a strange child, "Little boy; what's the matter with your face, little boy?"; and we know it is all over. To underline further both the extent of the disaster and its arbitrary, accidental nature, when the children return from their outing, before the effects of Eugenia's exposure are evident, Sir Hugh devises games for their further diversion, in the course of which he drops Eugenia from a raised plank. So that when she is taken with the infection, and when, some time later, is fortunate enough to recover from that disease —

though "seamed and even scarred by the horrible disorder," with "not a trace of her beauty left, no resemblance by which he could have known her" (bk. 1, chap. 3, p. 29) — it is discovered that she is not only permanently disfigured in feature by the smallpox but also permanently deformed in figure as a result of her fall from the plank! Eugenia, originally the most beautiful of the three Tyrold sisters, is now excluded from any possible participation in the beauty contest, which as a young woman without a large dowry is her best means of assuring herself a comfortable future. Life isn't fair, and Burney lets us know it in no uncertain terms!

Burney's fable here might almost seem to have been borrowed from the great sage of her day, Dr. Johnson, who was both an admirer of her fiction as well as a member of the circle of London intelligentsia to which Burney's father, a renowned musicologist, belonged. One of Johnson's popular *Rambler* essays of 1751 is a "letter" from a certain "Victoria" whose beauty, like Eugenia's, has been obliterated by the smallpox. But "Victoria," having lamented the loss of her beauty, records the advice of her "wise friend, Euphemia": "You have lost that which may indeed sometimes contribute to happiness, but to which happiness is by no means inseparably annexed. . . . Consider yourself, my Victoria, as a being born to know, to reason, and to act; rise at once from your dream of melancholy to wisdom and to piety; you will find that there are other charms than those of beauty, and other joys than the praise of fools."[5]

"Rise at once": and we may assume that the young woman thus addressed will do just that. There were many Victorias in the world in which Fanny Burney and Samuel Johnson lived. The woman afflicted with smallpox, whose value on the beauty-market is suddenly, *through no fault of her own*, rendered nil, is the extreme case of *any* ugliness, understood as an accident of nature rather than the result of some inner moral defect. And Eugenia too will, in the end, "rise" to the occasion. Near the close of the novel, she will announce to the world — and specifically to the men in it — that if she has suffered, the fault lies not in herself but in the misplaced value the opposite sex puts upon "external attractions" (bk. 10, chap. 14, p. 905). After such a recognition and such a speech, it seems only simple justice that Eugenia should win the heart and hand of one man who (albeit only after considerable time and some schooling) can see her inner merits and value *them*.

Told as I have just told it, through the bare delineation of its plot, Eugenia's story does indeed reinforce the Johnsonian moral. The cadenced tones in which she delivers her lecture on the "external attractions," however heartfelt the sentiment therein expressed, echo the formal intonations of Johnson's letter to Victoria. However, the story Burney actually gives us in the novel is much more complex than this outline suggests. The real moral of Burney's narrative, which we may read between the lines of the plot, or through its "subtext," is a different and more interesting one than Johnson's: it is that Eugenia's story doesn't, subjectively speaking, make sense. Eugenia's inner, subjective *experience* of ugliness is the story of a scrambled identity. This is the story of ugliness as I — and many other women, and men too — have experienced it.

We first sense the tension created by *Camilla*'s subtext in Sir Hugh's confused response to what he's done — which is, initially, a restatement (in his own cruder terms) of Johnson's dictum. If Eugenia cannot be the beautiful daughter, well then, he will see to it that she will be the rich daughter: he will make her, instead of Camilla, his heir. And he will make her the wise daughter too. He will nurture the scholarly inclinations already evident in the young child by hiring a tutor to give her a solid education in the classics. Rearing her at his own estate, he will also have educated abroad another ward, the young Clermont Lynmere, to be her future spouse. So all will come out well in the end, Sir Hugh assures himself. "For as to the mere loss of beauty, pretty as it is to look at, I hope it is no such great injury, as she'll have a splendid fortune, which is certainly a better thing, in point of lasting. For as to beauty, Lord help us! what is it? except just to the eye" (bk. 1, chap. 3, p. 33). But these words are no sooner out of his mouth than he discovers that his *feelings* are not quite so simple. Approaching his niece to embrace her, Sir Hugh "stopt and sighed involuntarily as he looked at her, saying: 'After all, she's not like the same thing! no more than I am myself. I shall never think I know her again, never as long as I live! I can't so much as believe her to be the same, though I am sure of its being true'" (ibid.). The alteration in Eugenia's outer appearance has, as the foolish but plain-speaking Sir Hugh dimly realizes, somehow changed *her*.

And how does Eugenia herself feel the change? Initially, she doesn't feel it at all. For Sir Hugh has issued strict orders that her "misfortune" never be alluded to in the household. "Those incidents, therefore, from never being named, glided imperceptibly from her thoughts; and she grew up as unconscious as she was innocent, that, though born with a beauty which surpassed that of her lovely sisters, disease and accident had robbed her of that charm ere she knew she possessed it" (bk. 1, chap. 7, p. 50). For the other members of the household, though, her misfortune has the quality of a guilty secret—something that's never supposed to be talked about but is constantly threatening to pop out of its hiding place. And eventually Eugenia too discovers the secret—significantly, just as she reaches the age of sexual maturation. But her discovery, coming when it does, suggests more than the social difficulties that may lie ahead for her (even though her spouse has already been chosen for her). Burney stages the scene brilliantly, in a half-finished house where Eugenia and Camilla find themselves abandoned, in the classic plight of the immured maiden, and here Eugenia's discovery of her ugliness feels to her like an exposure of her hidden sexual self—one which implies she is somehow deeply, inwardly, defective.

Eugenia and Camilla have been led by an ineffectual escort, a Mr. Dubster, to survey the country house he is having built for himself. Their protector disappears, and the two young women find themselves improbably marooned in the upper story of his unfinished house, unable to descend. The scene is a curious one, but it works emotionally because it recreates, in the social milieu of the eighteenth-century would-be gentleman, the timeless fable of the immured maiden, the helpless young virgin whose predicament inside a locked house (whether it be the site of her protection or her violation) teases us with the possibility of seduction. But here the seduction turns out to be a cruel mockery, or travesty, of the real thing.

The two abandoned girls cry out for help, but the only passersby are a group of country women, on their way to market, who, immediately noticing Eugenia's appearance, decide to have some sport with her. What does *she* have, they crudely inquire, that they should assist her? Trapped in the unfinished house, the sisters are indeed helpless; but the market-women taunt Eugenia with a deeper and more lasting powerlessness — her inability to arouse sexual desire, calling out with heavy sarcasm, "I suppose you think we'll sarve [serve, that is, assist] you for looking at? — no need to be paid?" "Yes, yes," says another, "Miss may go to market with her beauty; she'll not want for nothing if she'll shew her pretty face!" (bk. 4, chap. 3, p. 286). As women who deal in the realities of buying and selling, they know the value not only of their wares but of hers. And on a deeper level, they suggest that this violation, this parody of a rape, presently being enacted, is as close to the real thing as Eugenia will ever get. Which is, indeed, how she responds to their insults, sinking to the floor of the unfurnished chamber in a state of shock. Camilla tries to revive her by leaning over her and anxiously speaking on other subjects, "in hopes to dissipate a shock she was ashamed to console" (p. 288). *Ashamed*, because Camilla knows that on one level the market-women are exposing a guilty secret, the truth.

Eugenia feels the assault of this revelation as if it is something she hasn't known but should have known about herself all along — as if the interior, sexual part of herself has been exposed and discovered to be bad, ugly. She feels, that is, not merely what a disfigured young woman would feel, but what any girl, just coming of age, at some moments fears about herself — which is why the scene is so powerful. The market-women will, of course, be corrected: Eugenia's good father will dismiss their abuse as "the insolence of the hard-hearted, and ignorance of the vulgar" (bk. 4, chap. 5, p. 304). Which it is. But what Burney understands so well here, from Eugenia's point of view, is the depth of the injury to her sense of herself. Distraught, she criticizes the family members who, however well-intentioned, have been deceiving her all these years about herself, "assuring me I had nothing peculiar to myself, though I was so unlike all my family — of deluding me into utter ignorance of my unhappy defects, and then casting me, all unconscious and unprepared, into the wide world to hear them!" (bk. 4, chap. 4, p. 293). "I knew I was not handsome, but I supposed many people besides not handsome, and that I should pass with the rest . . . but the subject never seized my mind; I never reflected upon it at all, till abuse, without provocation, all at once opened my eyes, and *shewed me to myself!*" (ibid., 303, my italics). Then she shuts herself in her chamber, away from the world and from the members of her family who have thus betrayed her.

Hoping to console her and draw her out of her seclusion, her good father does just the *wrong* thing: he suggests that Eugenia might take a leaf from another contemporary moralist — in this case the leaf is drawn not from *The Rambler* but from the more popular *Spectator* essays of Addison and Steele. "Remember," he cautions her, "what Addison admirably says in one of the Spectators: 'A too acute sensibility of personal defects, is one of the greatest weaknesses of self-love'" (bk. 4, chap. 5, p. 302).[6] And at that remark, the ordinarily gentle child flies into a (dignified) rage: "I should be sorry, Sir, you should attribute to vanity what I now suffer. No! it is simply the effect of never hearing, never knowing, that so severe a call was to be made upon my fortitude, and therefore never arming myself to sustain it." What Burney shows us so clearly here, and where the import of her narrative (or *Camilla's* subtext) contradicts the superficial moralists' message, is that if Eugenia is to heal in spirit, what she needs is not *less* self-love but *more*.

Eugenia's father's ministrations are more successful on a subsequent occasion, when "straining her to his breast with the fondest parental commiseration, the tears, with which his eyes were over-

flowing, bedewed her cheeks" (bk. 4, chap. 5, p. 303). The consolatory power of the tear is far greater than that of the sermon — as
Eugenia's response makes clear: " 'O my father,' she cried, 'a tear
from your revered eyes afflicts me more than all else! Let me not
draw forth another, lest I should become not only unhappy, but
guilty. Dry them up, my dearest father — let me kiss them away.' "
The insult to Eugenia's appearances, as a personal, narcissistic injury, cannot be healed by the rejection of any part of herself, but
only by seeing her whole and loving her whole.[7]

Not surprisingly, Sir Hugh's elaborate scheme for Eugenia's
marriage goes awry. When young Clermont Lynmere, on whom
the classical education has not grafted as well as it has on Eugenia,
arrives in England to greet his intended bride, he rejects her on the
spot — or rather, not on the spot, because when Lynmere first sees
Eugenia it does not occur to him that *this* could be his destined
bride. (Sir Hugh, of course, has not given Lynmere any advance
notice of Eugenia's misfortune, ostensibly because it oughtn't to
matter, but really because he fears how much it may matter.) In another wonderfully moving and realistically rendered scene (bk. 7,
chap. 8, p. 561 — a chapter ironically titled "A Summons to Happiness"), on the afternoon of Lynmere's expected arrival, Eugenia,
rather than wait for him within doors, with Sir Hugh hovering over
her, decides to "take a stroll by herself in the park." She has been
instructed by her tutor "never to be unprovided with a book,"
and — just as I would have done in her situation! — she carries her
book with her. It will serve her in more than one way in this crisis.
On the most superficial level, the book provides a kind of camouflage, something she can hide behind if she needs to. It is also a dis-
traction, of the best sort — something meaningful but outside herself, in which she becomes absorbed while waiting for an event of
great personal moment to take place. And on a symbolic level the
book may serve as a reminder, to herself and perhaps also to Lynmere, that one cannot judge a book by its cover. In this last sense,
the book is a way of reminding Eugenia that should he reject her,
she has inner resources which may prove more valuable than this

union in the end. But what happens when Lynmere arrives is something Eugenia could not have anticipated. The young man walks
right by her without appearing to see her. In a few moments he returns and asks her whether she belongs to the house; he has been
told that one of the young ladies was this way, but can trace nobody. Has she perhaps seen any of them? Lynmere, it turns out,
has supposed his destined bride to be one of the maids! Her ugly
face is automatically processed by him as the equivalent of a servant's dress. The collapse Eugenia suffers here recapitulates the collapse following her encounter with the market-women, for again it
is a blow to her self-esteem. As an ugly young woman, to a pro-
spective mate, she is a person utterly without significance.

A woman's subjective experience of ugliness, as this scene so
nicely illustrates, exactly reverses her subjective experience of
beauty. Where the woman who knows herself as beautiful knows
herself the gratified object of the man's sexual curiosity, the ugly
woman defines herself (as Eugenia does here) by her failure to
arouse curiosity, by her invisibility. And such an antithesis, we may
notice, strikingly reverses the one we observed in the preceding
chapter. For the gazing man in the dominant patriarchal convention
it is precisely the beautiful woman who negates the impulse of curiosity and the ugly woman who (however uncomfortably) stim-
ulates it. This is not to suggest that men necessarily perceive woman's beauty one way, and women experience it in another. But it is,
I think, to suggest that the kind of "male gaze" a woman can honor
and enjoy — where the desire to discover her beauty is linked to a
desire to discover her otherness, both sexually and personally —
goes against a contrary tradition of masculine seeing deeply embedded in our culture.

Burney does not — as Dickens does in the same situation with
Esther Summerson in *Bleak House*[8] — sentimentalize by conferring
on the disfigured heroine at the end of the novel a fairy-tale beauty
that all (except the modest heroine herself) can see. What she does
do, when Melmond, the man Eugenia loves, finally realizes her
worth and takes her hand, is very suggestive. Having assured us that
"Eugenia once loved, was loved for ever," she goes on to say that

"where her countenance was looked at, her complexion was for-gotten; while her voice was heard, her figure was unobserved; where her virtues were known, they seemed but to be enhanced by her per-sonal misfortunes" (bk. 10, chap. 14, p. 912). It is the Johnsonian moral, but with a difference. The appeal to a beauty of "counte-nance" is an appeal to something seen; and the appeal to the beauty of Eugenia's voice confers on her an attraction within the world of sensory experience. The allusion to her "countenance" confirms an earlier moment in the novel, when Eugenia enters Camilla's cham-ber after having taken the self-sacrificing action of bestowing a large part of her fortune on Melmond so he can marry the vain and beautiful Indiana — which is what he then imagines he wants. "She entered with a bright beam upon her countenance, which, in defi-ance of the ravaging distemper that had altered her, gave it an expression almost celestial. It was the pure emanation of virtue, of disinterested, of even heroic virtue" (bk. 9, chap. 7, p. 754). Or, Burney implies, virtue *has* left its mark on Eugenia's features.

"Countenance" becomes a key term for those late eighteenth- and nineteenth-century women writers who do continue to present their heroines as beautiful — but on their own terms. For example, before we see her ourselves, we are told of the heroine of *Cœlebs in Search of a Wife*, an 1808 novel by the popular educator and moralist Hannah More, that the beauty of Lucilla Stanley "is that of *coun-tenance*: it is the stamp of mind intelligibly printed on the face. It is not so much the symmetry of features, as the joint triumph of in-tellect and sweet temper. A fine old poet [John Donne] has well de-scribed her: 'Her pure and eloquent blood / Spoke in her cheeks, and so distinctly wrought / That one could almost say her body thought.'"[9] And that is all we need to hear.

It is unfortunate that the term "countenance" is one which is all but lost to us today because it fixes so nicely just that point where inner nature and outer aspect intersect.[10] Our nearest equivalent, "expression," registers a more fleeting phenomenon: a benign "expression" on a face may cover a multitude of sins. But "coun-tenance" registers inner feeling, or temperament, at a deeper, more permanent level. It is what Kent is reading when he looks at the face

of King Lear, abused in his daughter's home, and vows to serve
him, saying, "You have that in your countenance which I would
fain call master . . . Authority" (act I, sc. 4, ll. 29–30). Lear's countenance expresses all his accumulated experience, everything that
has made him, for better or for worse, the man he is. "Countenance," then, is the marker of identity. And just as, over time, under extreme pressure or the impetus to grow and change, identity
may change, so will countenance change along with it. By the end
of the play Lear's countenance will no longer express authority, but
it may express something better — a wisdom painfully learned.[11]

In the heroine-portraiture of late eighteenth-century women's
fiction we also find a conscious rejection of the preliminary masculine interchange which prepares us to see the heroine as a collection of perfect parts. In a popular novel of 1791, *A Simple Story*,
Elizabeth Inchbald prepares us to see her heroine through a conversation, not between two men but two women. Though the
beauty question is by no means irrelevant here, Inchbald subtly prepares the woman who has not yet met Miss Milner — and her own
reader — to perceive her heroine's beauty through a new sort of
lens:

> "Is Miss Milner tall, or short?" again asked Mrs. Horton, fearing
> from the sudden pause which had ensued the subject should be
> dropped.
> "I don't know," answered Mrs. Hillgrave.
> "Is she handsome, or ugly?"
> "I really can't tell."
> "It is very strange you should not take notice!"
> "I did take notice, but I cannot depend upon my own judgment
> — to me she appeared as beautiful as an angel, but perhaps I was
> deceived by the beauties of her disposition."[12]

The speaker portrays the heroine here by refusing to portray in the
old terms. She avoids the set antitheses: tall or short, handsome or
ugly. She corrects her companion; for she has indeed "taken notice": "to me she appeared as beautiful as an angel." But she insists
on the subjectivity of her perception. She knows that her percep-

tion of Miss Milner's beauty is dependent on her perception of her internal qualities — or that beauty is the face of love.

The new heroine convention that emerges in women's fiction allows for a beauty that is often precisely unsettling rather than reassuring. This new way of seeing is played out, with amusing results, in *Pride and Prejudice* (1813). When Darcy first sees Elizabeth Bennet at the Netherfield ball, he says to his friend Bingley, "*You* are dancing with the only handsome girl in the room."[13] Bingley, who has fallen in love with Jane, replies, "Oh! she is the most beautiful creature I ever beheld! But there is one of her sisters sitting down just behind you, who is very pretty, and I dare say, very agreeable. Do let me ask my partner to introduce you." To which the aristocratic Darcy haughtily replies, in the evaluative mode of the patriarchal convention, "She is tolerable; but not handsome enough to tempt *me*; and I am in no humour at present to give consequence to young ladies who are slighted by other men. You had better return to your partner and enjoy her smiles, for you are wasting your time with me" (vol. 1, chap. 3, p. 12). What Darcy learns in the course of the novel is that this mode, so re-reinforcing of his own masculine sense of superiority (really just a high class version of the *Marty* "I got stuck with a dog" line) has nothing to do with genuine sexual attraction. And that discovery, because it demands an unsettling surrender to his own emotional vulnerability, is one that this proud man resists intensely. Austen wonderfully shows us — even as Darcy fights valiantly against it with all the verbal resources at his command — the resistance crumbling:

> Mr. Darcy had at first scarcely allowed her to be pretty; he had looked at her without admiration at the ball; and when they next met, he looked at her only to criticize. But no sooner had he made it clear to himself and his friends that she had hardly a good feature in her face, than he began to find it was rendered uncommonly intelligent by the beautiful expression of her dark eyes. To this discovery succeeded some others equally mortifying. Though he had detected with a critical eye more than one failure of perfect symmetry in her form, he was forced to acknowledge her figure to be

light and pleasing; and in spite of his asserting that her manners
were not those of the fashionable world, he was caught by their easy
playfulness.   *(vol. 1, chap. 6, pp. 21–22)*

Darcy's discovery here is not simply that a woman he had judged
inferior is, in fact, made of better stuff than he had first acknowledged. It is the discovery of a whole new way of seeing. Instead of
comparing Elizabeth to her sister Jane, he looks at *her*. And in
seeing her beauty, he sees the way her lively, intelligent spirit ani-
mates her whole person — and particularly her eyes. To Darcy it *is*
truly a "mortifying" discovery; and this is so not only because
Darcy is the sort of man who does not like to change his mind. It is
mortifying because what Darcy is really discovering here is his own
emotional susceptibility. And that is unsettling — to him especially
so — but also disturbing to all of us. The new feminine convention
of heroine-portraiture includes, as the patriarchal one does not, the
unsettledness that is part of the discovery of love. In terms of the
dynamics of sexual politics, it confers power on the sexual object
seen rather than restricting it to the one who does the seeing. It is
the man who is "caught" here, not the woman. But I do not want
to suggest that what we have in this new, women's convention is
simply a reversal of the old dynamic: the woman assuming power
over the man instead of the other way round. For this is a way of
seeing that is, ultimately, as liberating to the man as it is to the
woman, and that is the reason why in the end we are amused. We
have to smile at Darcy here (even if he can't smile at himself) because we know that what Darcy is seeing, and trying so hard not to
see, is what will free him.

A heroine, then, may still be beautiful, but she will have to have
a new kind of beauty, one which cannot be inventoried. We may
call it a "difficult" beauty, as it is difficult to apprehend in two
senses: difficult for us to perceive on the aesthetic level, and, on the
physical level, eluding the man's easy grasp. The absence of symmetry in Elizabeth Bennet's features, the insistence that her beauty
has its source in her inner personality (expressed in her eyes), the
"easy playfulness" of her manner, the mobility of her whole

person — all those elements which take Darcy by surprise and which keep her beauty in opposition to the static, predictable beauty of the woman of parts — are key features in the new women's convention of heroine-portraiture.

Austen's term for this whole cluster of qualities in its physical aspect is "prettiness." If "pretty" describes a lower level of beauty (in Johnson's *Dictionary*, "beauty without dignity, neat elegance without elevation"), it may also connote a beauty free of pretension. Austen's "pretty" heroines (even the shyest of them) inherit something of the attractiveness, the air of teasing come-uppance we find in that ubiquitous eighteenth-century creature, the "pretty fellow." Indeed, it is perhaps not irrelevant, in considering the "pretty" Austen heroine, to think all the way back to the original sense of the Old English "praetti3": "cunning, crafty, wily."[14] If her "pretty" heroines come in various shades of personality as well as of appearance, their rivals are invariably "handsome" women. The "handsome" woman is one with fine form or figure (usually in conjunction with full size or stateliness); but "handsome" women can also suggest "too much of a muchness."[15] In Humbert Humbert's idealization of the prepubescent Lolita, his darling's mother is dismissed as "that sorry and dull thing: a handsome woman."[16]

This is, essentially, how Austen portrays the "handsome" rival to her own "pretty" heroine — as the old woman of parts, seen now as *all too* predictable.[17] However virtuous (and no one, certainly, could be more virtuous than the "handsome" Jane Bennet in *Pride and Prejudice*), Austen's "handsome" woman is always condemned to play the *other* woman, the "pretty" woman's foil. Often an older sister or an older-sister surrogate, hers is the beauty that *can* be appraised by the judging man. Isabella Thorpe, in Austen's first novel, *Northanger Abbey* (written between 1798 and 1803, published posthumously in 1818), plays the foil to the emerging prettiness of that novel's "ugly duckling" heroine and is singled out from her own sisters as "the handsomest" of her own brood.[18] The Bertram sisters in *Mansfield Park* (1814), the showy foils to another neglected "ugly duckling" pretty heroine, are so handsome themselves as not to resent the arrival of another handsome woman (Mary Crawford) on the scene.[19] Mary Elliot in *Persuasion* (1816, published posthumously in 1818), another elder sister, at twenty-nine is "still the handsome Miss Elliot that she had begun to be thirteen years ago,"[20] as frozen and unchanging in spirit as in body. Emma Watson (in the early unfinished novel *The Watsons* (1804), is another "pretty" heroine with a "handsome" older sister.[21] In such a context it becomes all the more telling that one of Austen's greatest as well as her most disparate heroine — the "handsome" Emma Woodhouse of *Emma* (1816) — though technically a younger sister, lives the life of an only child (her sister being so much older than she). And it is Emma who is the recipient of the privileges as well as the authorial strictures that are the portion of Austen's "handsome" women.

Heroines in women's fiction (as heroes in men's) tend to be projections of their creator's own selves — and nowhere is this phenomenon more subtly, but perhaps importantly, felt than in the sense a writer projects onto her heroine of the feeling and texture of life as she herself has lived it, not only in the mind but in the body. (Such complex projections are the subject of chapters 3 and 4, on Charlotte Brontë and George Eliot, respectively.) So it is not surprising that as a young woman, and a younger sister, Jane Austen herself had something of the quixotic brightness she ascribes to a "pretty" heroine like Elizabeth Bennet. One acquaintance recalls her as the "prettiest, silliest, most affected husband-hunting butterfly."[22] Another recalls her as "pretty — certainly pretty . . . and a good deal of colour in her face — like a doll — no, that would not give at all the idea, for she had so much expression . . . very lively and full of humour . . ."[23] In a letter to her sister Cassandra, written in the year in which *Pride and Prejudice* was published, Austen says, speaking of the guests present at an evening's entertainment, "The Hammonds were there. Miss [the eldest daughter] looked very handsome, but I prefer her little, smiling, flirting sister Julia."[24] If Jane Austen herself was more like her pretty heroines, then it is all the more marvelous, and liberating, that in *Emma* she can allow us to see life, for once, through the eyes of the conventionally beautiful, privileged, and complacent young woman. The opening line of that novel declares, "Emma Woodhouse, handsome, clever, and rich, with a comfortable home and happy disposition, seemed to unite some of the best blessings of existence, and had lived nearly twenty-one years in the world with very little to distress or vex her." In *Emma* it is the unusual, unsettled and unsettling, socially disadvantaged young woman (Jane Fairfax) who must here play the part of the less likable, *other* woman.

In the ascendancy of the "pretty" heroine over her "handsome" rival we have a victory at once for women seen and valued finally for themselves and for the individualism we associate with the values of a rising economic class. Austen herself would have winced at our contemporary tendency to refer to her Elizabeth as a "middle-class" heroine: she is, after all, the daughter of a gentleman, and the pecuniary difficulties of the Bennet daughters — hence the urgency of their "capturing" husbands with money — are due to the entailment of their father's estate — the old younger-son problem. Still, in marrying "up" Elizabeth brings with her to the world of the aristocratic Darcy some of the qualities we associate with "bourgeois" egalitarianism.

Elizabeth wins the aristocratic Darcy's hand as a "pretty" girl, and keeps it as one. We know, that is, that Elizabeth, as mistress of Pemberly, will remain Elizabeth; she will continue to question her husband's assumptions about rank and order; she will continue to laugh at life (even though she may never succeed in getting her husband to laugh at himself); her eyes will not lose their look of sparkling, questioning, intelligent beauty. Compare Elizabeth's fate with that of Pamela, the heroine of Samuel Richardson's 1740 novel. Pamela *wins* her master, Mr. B, as a "pretty" girl — "Every body talks how you have come on . . . and some say you are very pretty;[25] "She told me I was a pretty wench" (letter 4, p. 8); "for, he said, I was very pretty"(letter 6, p. 11); "it is no wonder he should love you, you are so pretty; though so much beneath him" (letter 8, p. 37). But when Mr. B introduces his "pretty rustic" to the assembled gentry, she is greeted in terms appropriate for a lord's bride-to-be: she is now, in the evaluative terms of the patriarchal convention, "the loveliest maiden in England" and "fair excellence" (p. 299).[26] Most telling is that, on the morning of her wedding, Pamela herself draws attention to Mr. B's use of the new nomenclature: "Indeed, sir, said I, I have been reading over the solemn service. And what thinks my fairest (for so he called me) of it?" (pp. 358–59). From this point on, Pamela is always the fairest maid of the patriarchal convention: "in the beauty of your person, you excel all the ladies I ever saw" (p. 370); she is to her betrothed now repeatedly, "my fairest" (pp. 377, 387) and "my fair-one" (p. 429). In taking on *his* definition of her beauty with his name and rank, Pamela is giving up her own identity. This is precisely the fate that Elizabeth Bennet does not choose in her union with the desirable, aristocratic man.

The very first thing we hear about Elizabeth Bennet in *Pride and Prejudice* is that she is "not half so handsome" as her sister Jane. But the words come to us from Mrs. Bennet—and after reading just two pages of *Pride and Prejudice* we know enough about that maternal figure to know how to value her estimate. Just as Elizabeth Bennet's "prettiness" is defined through contrast with the "handsomeness" of her elder sister, Jane, so everywhere in the new women's convention, the new, unsettling, preemptive beauty can only be defined by placing it against the background of the old, reassuring kind. Gradually, this new way of portraying beauty becomes as much a convention—that is to say, a shared vision which expresses shared attitudes toward life—as the patriarchal convention of beauty. To take just one, relatively early example, in Fanny Burney's *Camilla* (1796), the heroine is at the start conceded to be not "half so great a beauty" as her rival, Indiana (bk. 1, chap. 1, p. 11). Then in a later scene, an elaborate set-piece, Burney develops the contrast between the attractions of the two young women. Indiana's beauty is defined as that which cannot disappoint (note the use of negative praise), while Camilla's beauty "though neither perfect nor regular," takes "even judgment itself, the coolest and last betrayed of our faculties . . . by surprise, though it was not till she was absent the seizure was detected" (bk. 2, chap. 4, p. 84). Such pairings become so commonplace by the mid nineteenth century that when we hear, for instance, on the opening page of Elizabeth Gaskell's 1855 novel, *North and South*, of the striking beauty of the sleeping Edith, which all through the childhood of the two cousins had "been remarked upon by everyone,"[27] we know that it is not Edith but the unobserved, unremarked-upon Margaret who will be the novel's heroine. Similarly, when in Harriet Martineau's *Deerbrook* (1839) the general voice acclaims, "How very handsome Hester is," and "It is rather odd that one sister should have all the beauty. . . . I do not see anything striking in Margaret,"[28] we know some correction is in order.

Heroines of *difficult* beauty come in all shapes and sizes. She may be tall or short, dark or fair, robust or delicate—just so long as the overall effect is to force us to rethink our preconceived categories. If there *is* any physical predictor for the style of beauty or body-type which marks these heroines, we might say that theirs is the "unfashionable" style of beauty which is *just becoming* fashionable. Thus in the latter half of the nineteenth century the large, unruly dark-haired woman tends to replace the delicate blonde of the thirties and forties, who has herself supplanted some years earlier the tall, elegant beauty of the Regency period. "I would have darkened and smoothed my Kirsteen's abundant hair if I could," says the popular novelist, Margaret Oliphant, of her 1890 heroine, "for in those days nobody admired it,"[29] making it clear that her turn-of-the-century reader is more perspicacious. In this connection we may note that Charlotte Brontë's conspicuously small heroines and George Eliot's conspicuously large ones, even as they are the extensions of their creators' own selves, are also exaggerations rather than distortions of current, that is, the new, fashion. The woman writer does not want to make it too easy for us to see her heroine's beauty; but she does not want to make it impossible either!

When we think of our bodies being really seen, we are apt to think of them being seen accurately and in detail. One recalls all those jokes in which the wife asks the husband what she was wear-

ing on a certain memorable occasion, or perhaps even what color
her eyes are, and he reveals his uncaringness by giving the wrong
answer. But in life and in art I'm not sure that verisimilitude is really
the issue — though curiosity certainly is. What counts is not *what* is
seen (how much or how little, how precisely or imprecisely) but
how it is seen — whether the body is seen with a desire for mastery
or with the eyes of love. The person who says, "how beautiful you
look," may be saying something more truly noticing than the one
who remembers the exact pattern of the print on the dress you
wore. Thus the irregular features which become so frequent a mark
of the heroine in women's fiction in the mid nineteenth-century do
not speak for an observer who is looking at a "real" woman rather
than at a stereotyped one. It is a mistake to suppose that the crucial
difference between the portraits in the patriarchal convention and
those in the new convention of difficult beauty is that the one is
vague and overly stylized where the other is rich in concrete, realistic detail.[30] All seeing stylizes: what matters is the meaning that
informs a given stylization.

This new convention of "difficult" beauty, invented by women
novelists, is not the exclusive property of writers of that sex. As
women often see their bodies in the compartmentalizing, deper-
sonalizing way that men do, so do men often see women's bodies
as women would wish them to be seen, without dehumanizing
them. And male novelists, who wish to portray the bodies of their
heroines thus, "borrow" the women's convention of portraiture I
have been analyzing in this chapter.[31] Of those who do so, the
nineteenth-century novelist Anthony Trollope is, I think, the outstanding example. Mary Thorne in *Dr. Thorne* (1858) and Lucy
Morris in *The Eustace Diamonds* (1873) are both presented as "difficult" beauties. Eleanor Harding in *The Warden* (1857) is another
example — and a particularly interesting one — because Trollope
does something here that would be difficult for a woman novelist
to do: he registers and legitimizes an interplay between a woman's
desire to *make* herself attractive in her lover's eyes and her desire to
simply, effortlessly, *be* so. Women have so often been accused of

using their beauty that a woman writer may well feel that any acknowledgment of contrivance, or even any acknowledgment that
a woman is conscious of her beauty's effect, impugns her integrity.
But here Trollope knows better. He presents a typical "difficult
beauty" portrait of Eleanor, as she is seen by her lover, John Bold,
at a crucial moment in the plot: she has come to persuade him to
bend his strict rules to help her father, whom (as a matter of prin-
ciple) Bold has done out of a job. "How beautiful Eleanor appeared
to him," Trollope begins, and follows up with the usual concessions: hers is not a perfect beauty, her sister is generally agreed to be
prettier, she must be seen aright to be properly appreciated. Then
Trollope does something new. He interrupts the lover's portrait to
take us back to the scene of Eleanor's preparation for this interview,
in which we see her "getting herself up" for it.

> Eleanor was certainly thinking more of her father than herself as
> she arranged her hair before the glass and removed the traces of sor-
> row from her face. And yet I should be untrue if I said that she was
> not anxious to appear well before her lover. Why else was she so
> sedulous with that stubborn curl that would rebel against her hand,
> and smooth so eagerly her ruffled ribands? Why else did she damp
> her eyes to dispel the redness, and bite her pretty lips to bring back
> the color? Of course she was anxious to look her best, for she was
> but a mortal angel after all. But had she been immortal, had she flit-
> ted back to the sitting-room on a cherub's wings, she could not have
> had a more faithful heart, or a truer wish to save her father at any
> cost to herself.[32]

It is a wonderfully understanding moment, and Trollope's tone of
knowingness comes from his understanding that Eleanor's impulses are, on the deepest level, all of a piece. Her desire to appeal
to John Bold's sense of what is due to her father, as a decent and a
suffering man, is not really at odds with her desire to encourage, in
the most forceful way she can, his desire for a union with herself.

In choosing a "difficult" beauty over an "easy" one, women
novelists are not doing something male novelists never do; nor are
they inventing a whole new aesthetic. What is new is the use they

make of a vision of beauty that is, in fact, central to the aesthetic discourse of the age. The distinction these writers are making between two ways of looking at women's beauty is, in essence, the same distinction Edmund Burke formulates in 1756 about beauty in general in his famous treatise, *A Philosophical Inquiry into the Sublime and the Beautiful*. Burke terms "the beautiful" all experiences which inspire feelings of tenderness, peace, and calm. The beautiful, for Burke, implies susceptibility: what is beautiful to the touch, for instance, is that which offers little resistance.[33] The sublime, on the other hand, inspires feelings of awe, discomposure, even fear. But where Burke locates our response to feminine attractiveness on one side of this great divide — "The beauty of women is considerably owing to their weakness or delicacy . . . (section 24) — Burney and the other women writers we are looking at locate it on the other side, as an aspect of "the sublime," as an experience which even as it is ultimately confirming, is also unsettling, driven by curiosity, a desire to penetrate the unknown.

Fairy tales, as Bruno Bettelheim has taught us to understand, often give expression to and suggest a resolution of a child's deepest, hidden anxieties.[34] We may find a confirmation for the meaning these women novelists bring to the discovery of their heroines' beauty in the fairy tale that deals most explicitly with the discovery of beauty, as a woman may experience it — *Cinderella*. It is the very fairy tale most often cited by feminists as an example of a patriarchal culture's schooling of girl children for a life of subservience to men. The usual feminist reading of *Cinderella* is that it defines success for the young girl in terms of victory in the beauty contest: she wins the Prince by appearing as the most beautiful woman at the ball and (to reinforce the message) by proving that she has the smallest foot of any woman in the kingdom. The latter form of comparative evaluation, especially if this particular motif comes to us from an oriental version of the story, as it may, implies that what immobilizes a woman is the very thing that makes her desirable.[35] But I would read this fairy tale differently. First of all, as Bettelheim points out,[36]

Cinderella is a much feistier girl in the Grimm version of the story (closer to the many versions of this most widely diffused of all fairy tales) than she is in the prettified version of the late-seventeenth-century French courtier, Charles Perrault, with which thanks to Walt Disney, we are likely to be more familiar. The Grimm Cinderella does not accept her degraded position in her stepmother's household graciously, but performs the most menial of household chores only under compulsion. Superficially, her appearance has changed — "they took to calling her Ashputtle (or 'Cinder-ella') because she always looked dusty and dirty."[37] But Cinderella knows, deep in her heart, that she does not deserve her degraded state: she is really better, more beautiful, than her stepsisters. That assurance comes to her, significantly, from the sustenance of her relationship with her dead mother, whose grave she waters daily with her tears. And the agent of her redemption is no magical fairy godmother with a pumpkin coach but the spirit of that same mother. So, even though the knowledge may be precarious, as it is threatened by her present status, Cinderella still retains a sense of herself as a beautiful, loved child. When the time comes for the great ball, this Cinderella does not cheerfully assist her stepsisters in their preparations; she begs to be allowed to attend the ball herself. Her request is, of course, refused; but the point is, she has not given up on herself; she feels entitled to be taken seriously as a sexually eligible young woman. And when she does get there, she can cast off the Ashputtle disguise and appear to the Prince as the beautiful young woman she truly is. Furthermore, the Grimm Cinderella leaves the ball, not at her mentor's bidding, but by her own choice — thus forcing the Prince to seek her out, and meet her on her own terms. Bettelheim suggests that Cinderella may need to have the Prince see and accept the bad as well as the good side of herself.[38] All children (and, we might add, many adults) fear they may not be loved because of the angry, jealous, bad feelings they keep hidden within themselves. Maybe they really are bad and *deserve* the ugliness that has been thrust upon them. This, of course, is precisely the fear that Burney's Eugenia struggles with; and the anxiety is re-

solved in both stories in essentially the same way — by having those
the Cinderella figure loves come to her, and assure her of her
desirability.

There is yet another sense, I think, in which the Prince's coming to Cinderella and discovering that the lost slipper fits *her* foot,
may feel like a confirmation of her identity. For the Prince is not
only saying here that he has finally found the most beautiful woman in the kingdom (the one with the smallest foot); he is saying
he has found the *same* woman, the one he danced with and fell
in love with at the ball. A shoe, we know, will never fit another
foot so well as the one for which it was made. In the Grimm version that fact is nicely brought out by the stepsisters' gruesome mutilation of their feet in a desperate effort to squeeze them into
the too-small shoe, and cheat Cinderella out of her prize. ("Never
mind," their practical mother assures each in turn; when you get
to be queen, you won't need to walk anymore!" [p. 88]). It is the
stepsisters, then, not Cinderella, who act out the role of the sub-
servient, self-mutilating woman. The shoe slips onto Cinderella's
foot effortlessly: she will not have to constrain herself to assume
her new role as the Prince's bride. In that effortless slipping on
of the shoe there is certainly also the promise of an equally neat sexual fit between the Prince and Cinderella. And here again, the man's
delighted discovery of the woman's beauty is the discovery of her
sexual parts — not as disembodied objects but as a part of her own
unique self, to be accepted and loved.

Recent feminist criticism would suggest that a woman who resists knowing herself as beautiful is making a brave act of self-
assertion: by choosing not to be beautiful she is, in effect, opting out
of the patriarchal society, refusing to play the game. Such an analysis may be too simple though. If we think of ugliness as the expression of a latent fear that one may not be good in one's inner self, then
the ugly woman may be denying rather than asserting herself. Such
a form of denial is, I think, fairly common among adolescent girls,
whose feelings about their own sexuality are almost bound to be
somewhat ambivalent. I remember that, as an adolescent myself,

though I longed to be told that I was beautiful, when that did happen it was in a context that made me uncomfortable. My father would tell me, on certain formal occasions, that I looked beautiful — almost as beautiful, he would say, as my mother had been. This was, of course, meant as a compliment, and to some extent felt like one. Any comparison with my dead, exalted, but only dimly remembered mother, coming from my father, was the highest praise. But while (like Cinderella) I wanted to know my own beauty through a link with my mother, I also felt that, as my father's compliment implied, the comparison with my dead mother was one that would always define me as second best. After all, my mother's beauty (in part, no doubt, just because she was no longer living), like all her other assets, had been elevated to something very close to goddess status. More importantly, though I don't think I was aware of the fact at the time, I probably really wanted to be seen as beautiful, not just in terms of that comparison, but in my own right. And it occurs to me that one reason I may have remained plain all through the period of my adolescence, or through the period when I was still living at home, was that it felt safe. It felt safer, that is, to be plain than to enter into an unacknowledged competition with my dead mother. It was only when I got to college and began to meet men in a context outside the family setting, that I began to feel myself as someone who might be attractive to men. And it's been hard, I realize, to maintain a balance between wanting to identify myself with my mother — wanting to look like her, liking those pictures in which I can see the resemblance between us — and wanting to feel attractive on my own terms. For, though I can see a resemblance between us in certain images, in fact I do not have her "classic" beauty, but something else, a certain look I see more of in the pictures of the women in my father's family, and then something else too, something that's just me!

The idea that the beauty of a heroine might not simply be difficult for another person (particularly for a potential lover, perhaps) to recognize, but that it might be difficult for the heroine herself to assume — what we might call the motif of the heroine's *becoming beautiful* — is prominent in the fiction of nineteenth-century women writers. Jane Austen's Fanny Price, for one, the heroine of *Mansfield Park* (published in 1814), certainly knows the consolations of plainness, particularly valuable in a poor relation. At the opening of that novel the elder members of the wealthy Bertram family are debating whether to bring the ten-year-old Fanny, a product of Mrs. Bertram's sister's unfortunate marriage, into their own home, to be raised alongside their own daughters and (eligible) sons, a proposition not without risk from their point of view. "I don't say she would be so handsome as her cousins," says another resident Bertram sister reassuringly, "I dare say she would not" (vol. 1, chap. 1, p. 8). And Fanny, when first met, is obligingly plain — though we may note the hint of a new-convention beauty, in the "prettiness of countenance," which comes out when she takes the initiative of speaking, at the end of this portrait. Fanny is seen, significantly, not by an omniscient narrator — and in fact Austen *never* presents beauty in anything other than subjective terms[39] — but through the eyes of the appraising Bertrams, who have their own interest in the subject in question: "Fanny Price was at this time just ten years old, and though there might not be much in her first appearance to captivate, there was, at least, nothing to disgust her relations. She was small of her age, with no glow of complexion, nor any other striking beauty; exceedingly timid and shy, and shrinking from notice; but her air, though awkward, was not vulgar, her voice was sweet, and when she spoke, her countenance was pretty" (vol. 1, chap. 2, p. 12).

Here it is not the man, as in *Pride and Prejudice*, who has to learn to discover the heroine's prettiness: it is the heroine herself. And Fanny is not at all sure that she wants to give up the safety of her dependent, asexual status in the Bertram household. She has gotten used to living in the room without a fire, taking care of her hypochondriacal aunt, and playing the piano while the others dance. It is Edmund, the elder Bertram son — it can only be Edmund, whom Fanny loves — who begins to talk her out of it, trying to persuade Fanny that she "must harden [her]self to the idea of being worth looking at . . . must try not to mind growing up into a pretty woman" (vol. 2, chap. 3, p. 154). Edmund is being partly facetious here — he is also discovering his own love for Fanny, in presenting to her "her uncle's estimate of her charms." But Fanny — or a part of her — really does mind being looked at and really is afraid of assuming a sexual identity and a life of her own, which will mean (inevitably) having the guts to defy her patrons. Whether Fanny ever really does stop minding it, whether she ever does fully *know herself,* as others know her, as a fully sexual, "pretty" Austen heroine, is not entirely clear. What is important for my purposes, is that for Fanny to say "yes" to Edmund, is an act of self-assertion. And in that act of self-assertion, she becomes beautiful — in his eyes at least. Moreover, if Fanny wins out over Mary in Edmund's heart ultimately because she is the more virtuous woman of the two, Austen carefully avoids setting up the contest in Edmund's mind as one between Fanny's virtue and Mary's beauty. Or, ever sensitive to the complex workings of sexual desire, she shows the better woman *becoming,* in the eyes of a worthy lover, the more desirable one: ". . . what was there now to add, but that he should learn to prefer soft light eyes to sparkling dark ones — And being always with her, and always talking confidentially, and his feelings exactly in that favorable state which a recent disappointment gives, those soft light eyes could not be very long in obtaining the preeminence" (vol. 3, chap. 17, p. 367). Austen is smiling at her lovers here. But she is not suggesting that Edmund's vision is distorted or narrowed when he comes to prefer Fanny's soft light eyes to Mary's sparkling dark ones. The thrust of the passage is ultimately to enlarge rather than diminish our sense of life's possibilities. That our subjective vision — the only kind we have — should be able to make beautiful the object of our love is a wonderful fact of human perception.

Like Fanny Price in *Mansfield Park,* Anne Elliot in *Persuasion,* Austen's last finished novel, has to *learn* to see herself as a pretty, sexually eligible woman. Anne's reluctance is that of the incipient spinster rather than the orphan-child. For Anne at twenty-six (as perhaps for the once "pretty," "husband-hunting," but now ailing

Jane Austen at thirty) prettiness seems to lie not before but behind her: "A few years before, Anne Elliot had been a very pretty girl, but her bloom had vanished early; and as even in its height, her father had found little to admire in her (so totally different were her delicate features and mild dark eyes from his own), there could be nothing in them, now that she was faded and thin, to excite his esteem" (vol. 1, chap. 1, p. 11).

Where Fanny is a poor girl, hesitant to "capture" a wealthy man, Anne is a wealthy woman, whose romantic choice — that of a sea captain — is below rather than above her own position on the social ladder. The opposition to the match comes from her world rather than from his: it is Anne's own "handsome" relations who frown on this alliance. And yet, like Fanny's, Anne's plainness comes out of her willing victimization by others' narcissistic desires. At nineteen Anne had let herself be "persuaded" to give up a love match, and in doing so, she has lost her looks. As Sir Elliot sees it,

> Elizabeth [the eldest daughter] had succeeded, at sixteen, to all that was possible, of her mother's rights and consequence; and being very handsome, and very like himself, her influence had always been great, and they had gone on together most happily. His two other children were of very inferior value. Mary had acquired a little artificial importance, by becoming Mrs. Charles Musgrove; but Anne, with an elegance of mind and sweetness of character, which must have placed her high with any people of real understanding, was nobody with either father or sister: her word had no weight; her convenience was always to give way — she was only Anne. *(ibid.)*

Anne does regain her prettiness, and a fuller celebration of her sexuality than Fanny, with the recovery of love. Her beauty is restored in Lyme, where Anne is away from the baleful influence of her father at Kellynch Hall and is reunited with Wentworth, her lover, in a seaside setting that suggests nature's regenerative powers and also her lover's life as a sea captain, with all its exciting hazards. Here Anne can begin to let herself fall in love again — and regain her lost beauty. Pleased as we are at Anne's recovery, we may note in passing that there is no question of Wentworth's appearance having been altered beyond *her* recognition, by a corresponding grief at their long separation. He has been too busy, too active in the pursuit of his chosen career, in those seven years to grieve over a lost love. Anne, on the contrary, has had little to do in those same years but to feel it, and to lose her looks. This is one of many differences *Persuasion* records, in a narrative voice that is truthful and passionate and never shrill, between the life-experiences of women and men in Austen's era — perhaps one that still has relevance to our own.

In a charming bit of dialogue, close to the end of *Persuasion*, the reunited lovers are engaged in the delightful ritual of rehearsing all the misadventures and misunderstandings which have kept them apart for so long. Wentworth recalls a recent conversation with his brother, after he and Anne had become reacquainted but before there was (at least on his part) any question of a renewed love between them. His brother had then inquired "if you were personally altered, little suspecting that to my eye you could never alter" (vol. 3, chap. 11, p. 231). Now Anne knows that in making this assertion Wentworth is not being quite honest, or is not quite accurately remembering his sentiments of only a few months past: for he had found her — as her sister, overhearing the remark, had gone out of her way to inform Anne — "so altered he would not have known [her]," and she has not forgotten that remark. But now "Anne smiled, and let it pass." In her silent smiling she is very much an Austen heroine; a Brontë heroine or an Eliot one would have wanted more from her lover — not more words necessarily, but more truth. But what Anne feels, Austen goes on to explain, is that "It was too pleasing a blunder for a reproach. It is something for a woman to be assured, in her eight-and-twentieth year, that she has not lost one charm of earlier youth; but the value of such homage was inexpressibly increased to Anne by comparing it with former words, and feeling it to be the result, not the cause of a revival of his warm attachment" (vol. 3, chap. 11, p. 231).

Anne can enjoy the compliment, knowing it to be untrue both to the reality of her appearance and to Wentworth's earlier perception of it. The compliment is pleasing, and Austen will not deny her heroine the pleasure of gratified vanity. But the real pleasure comes from Anne's understanding of why Wentworth should now say "to my eye you could never alter" — because he is seeing her now through the eyes of love. And Anne smiles too because she knows, as Wentworth does not, that in beauty, as in love, one never does get it *all* back. She has recovered her prettiness, but it is not the prettiness of the inexperienced girl of nineteen who fell in love with Captain Wentworth. Anne Elliot at twenty-eight has "every beauty excepting bloom" (vol. 2, chap. 5, p. 146) — the feature which was so conspicuous a part of Jane Austen's own prettiness,[40] and which she knew herself losing in 1816, when she wrote *Persuasion*, in failing health at the age of forty-one, in what was to be the penultimate year of her short life. Jane Austen was not as fortunate as Anne Elliot in respect to love: the young man with whom she had fallen in love at the age of twenty never returned to her after their union was prevented by a family whose plans for the young Tom Lefroy (and perhaps his own plans as well) did not include marriage with a portionless daughter of a clergyman.

But if Austen *had* given her heroine back her youthful "bloom," she would have weakened the contrast between Anne and her "handsome" father and sister whose feelings, like their faces, are impervious to change. Moreover, in giving her heroine back a beauty with every charm *but* bloom, Austen is insisting all the more forcefully that the marriage between Anne and Wentworth now is one they make themselves. So, again, becoming beautiful and realizing fully one's identity, claiming one's right to a life of one's own choosing, are united.

I want to look at one more fictional example of what we might call the "becoming beautiful" motif in nineteenth-century women's fiction because it hints at an even more profound reason why a young woman might feel anxiety about letting go of her asexual, or plain, status. My model here is Molly Gibson in Elizabeth Gaskell's wonderful last novel, *Wives and Daughters*, published serially between 1864 and 1866. Like so many heroines of Victorian fiction,

Molly Gibson is a young girl who has lost her mother in her early childhood, and thus has to find her own way toward her adult female sexuality. In Molly's case, however, the father is not a self-absorbed Sir Elliot but a devoted and hard-working doctor, whom Molly adores, and who is deeply attached to his only child. But, as Molly approaches sexual maturity and "unsuitable" young men begin paying her attention, Mr. Gibson decides that his daughter needs a mother. (Little is said here — perhaps significantly — about his own sexual needs.) In any case, he makes a poor choice. The new Mrs. Gibson, self-absorbed and materialistic, doesn't stand a chance of winning Molly's affection — not that she tries hard to gain it. Molly's anxiety about her own physical attractiveness comes out, significantly, on the day of her father's wedding. She is wearing a dress picked out for her by her new "mamma." "I wonder if I'm pretty, thought she. I almost think I am — in this kind of dress I mean, of course.'" As she descends the stairs, "and with sly blushes presented herself for inspection, she was greeted with a burst of admiration. 'Well, upon my word! I shouldn't have known you,' says one family friend; and another observes, 'Well, my dear, if you were always dressed, you would be prettier than your dear mamma, whom we always reckoned so very personable'" (chap. 13, p. 187). But Molly, in this guise, can't "know herself" either: the primal wish that *she* be first in her father's affection would then be too near the surface of her consciousness. So she retreats into the protective cover of plainness — or sexual immaturity. When the novel's eligible young man meets Molly, all he sees is "a badly-dressed, and rather awkward girl, with black hair and an intelligent face, who might help him in the task he had set himself of keeping up a bright general conversation during the rest of the evening" (chap. 8, p. 119). Molly achieves sexual invisibility again — which is what she thinks she wants. I might, incidentally, observe that though Eugenia's "guilty secret" has no rational basis, it could be read as a displacement of her sister Camilla's guilty secret, which is the same as Molly's is here — an Oedipal attachment to her father. If the secret is displaced in the earlier novel from the heroine to her sister, perhaps that's because Gaskell is conscious of what Molly's plainness is all about, and Burney is not conscious of the source of her heroine's anxieties.

In any case, having assumed the part for a good reason, Molly plays the role of the virtuous daughter well; she even helps her new stepsister Cynthia (the old "picture-book" beauty, the undisputed victor in the beauty contest) win Roger's love. Eventually, though, Molly's virtue takes its toll upon her constitution; she becomes gravely ill. And in her illness and recovery she makes the symbolic transition from girlhood to womanhood that, on the deepest level, she really wants to make. When she next sees Roger, after his long absence, he discovers her beauty, for now Molly can become beautiful: "'Osborne [his elder brother] was right!' said he. 'She has grown into delicate fragrant beauty, just as he said she would'" (chap. 55, p. 648). And now that she is ready for him, Roger can discover his love for her.

Wives and Daughters is not quite finished — Gaskell died before completing it — but we don't need the missing final chapter. All we need to hear (after the complications of his entanglement with Cynthia have been disposed of) is that Roger "hardly recognized [Molly], although he acknowledged her identity. He began to feel that admiring deference which most young men experience when conversing with a very pretty girl; a sort of desire to obtain her good opinion in a manner very different to his old familiar friendliness" (chap. 58, p. 672). We end with the physical attraction which includes, as it always does, some element of irrational idealization. And if Roger does not immediately recognize this new Molly, she now *can* know herself, as she could not before, as a beautiful woman.

In another favorite fairy tale, *The Ugly Duckling*, where the "becoming beautiful" motif is played out, we can see — with the transparency of the fairy tale's mode, the connection we have seen in all these realistic fictions between becoming sexually mature and becoming more fully oneself. *The Ugly Duckling* is not a fairy tale in the classic sense that *Cinderella* is — an orally transmitted story of which there are numerous variant versions in different countries. *The Ugly Duckling* is a literary creation, a story written for children by a particular individual at a particular time: Hans Christian Andersen, who wrote in the mid-nineteenth century. Its authorship is particularly relevant, since Andersen knew himself as an ugly man. (Among other things, Andersen's story may remind us that beauty and ugliness are not just problems for women.)

Like all fairy tales, and most fictions, *The Ugly Duckling* has a consolatory, or affirmative, message. The message is, on one level, a lesson in the fallacy of judging on the basis of what one sees in a limited world. The ugly duckling only seems ugly because he is reared in the wrong community: he is like the black girl, Pecola, who has the misfortune to be labeled "ugly" because she lives in a world where whites are dominant and therefore beautiful. The world of the Ugly Duckling (as, often, our own) is a very small one. " 'Do you think this is the whole world?' said the mother. 'It stretches all the way to the other side of the garden, right into the parson's meadow. But I've never been there!' "[42] That the ugly duckling *is* ugly at the moment of his birth is presented as a simple fact: "He was very big and ugly" — since that is how he appears to the mother duck who has just hatched him as one of her own. Misclassified as a duckling, his largeness has to be read as ugliness. " 'Now that's a terribly big duckling!' she said. 'None of the others looks like that!' " (p. 137). The message to the child reading the story is that he too may be misclassified, out of place, reared in the wrong company. Once he frees himself from the confined world of the ducks and finds out what he really is — a swan — he will be recognized as beautiful. And there is the added comfort for the ugly duckling child of knowing that, on an absolute scale, swans are much more beautiful than ducks!

But there is another message in *The Ugly Duckling* story. For it is only when he meets the swans that, in a sense, the Ugly Duckling *becomes* himself a swan. Up until that point he is only a swan in potential. Andersen has nicely timed the events of the narrative so that the interval between the Ugly Duckling's birth (in the spring) and his wanderings (through the long, cold winter), until his meeting with the swans (in the following spring) coincides with the time-span of a swan's maturation. As a cygnette the swan is "a clumsy grayish-black bird," in effect, an ugly duckling. Only when he matures does he acquire the beautiful white plumage and the grace we associate with the swan. In Andersen's story the moment when the Ugly Duckling is himself seen by the company of swans is the same moment that he himself becomes a swan: " 'Just kill me,' said the poor creature, and bowed down his head toward the surface of the water and awaited his death. But what did he see in the clear water? Under him he saw his own reflection, but he was no longer a clumsy, grayish-black bird, ugly and disgusting. He was a swan himself!" (p. 146). Beauty, then, is not simply in the eye of the beholder; it may take time, as long as it takes to fully realize one's own sexual maturity, to know oneself as beautiful.

Beauty as the confirmation of one's identity, the outward expression of an inner reality: beauty as the face of love. As I said in my introductory chapter, this is how I would *like* to see it; it is how the eighteenth- and nineteenth-century women novelists I've been discussing have helped me to see beauty. But it isn't how I always, in fact, experience beauty. And there is one novel, by a twentieth-century woman writer, who both is and is not the heir to the novelists I've been discussing in this chapter, that I find myself returning to and feeling unsettled by because it forces me to think of beauty in the *other* way: beauty as a gift, arbitrarily conferred; beauty as privilege — and ugliness, then, as unfairness, as a disadvantage one may just be stuck with. The novel is Margaret Drabble's first one, *A Summer Bird-Cage* (published in 1963), written when Drabble was in her mid-twenties. When I came upon it at the same age, I found it both riveting and disturbing. Drabble's heroine is a young woman with whom I felt a good deal of kinship. Privileged socially and economically, energetic and "serious," Sarah is, as I was then, the possessor of "a lovely, shiny, useless new degree."[43] As I did, she yearns for all the truly meaningful things in life: "leaves and flowers and fruit" (work, love, children, friends). Not being ruthless, like her older sister Louise, or even particularly self-assertive, Sarah hasn't much of an idea of how she's going to get it all. And, as I did, she feels very uneasy about the beauty question. She knows she's not a "knock-out beauty," like Louise (an older sister in the tradition of the nineteenth-century, prettier-but-perhaps-not-really-so-beautiful-after-all sister). And Sarah feels strangely, obsessively, haunted by the specter of a decidedly unattractive cousin, with whom she both does and does not identify herself: "I was always one for seeing things in extremes, and because I wasn't as beautiful as Louise I assumed I was as plain as Daphne; whereas in fact if there is a barrier down the middle of mankind dividing the sheep from the goats I am certainly on Louise's side of it as far as physical beauty goes" (chap. 2, p. 21). Most of the time Sarah feels herself on the Louise side of the barrier, "as far as physical beauty goes." What Daphne inspires in her — at Louise's wedding, for instance, where Daphne looks "a total fright" in the ultra-smart bridesmaid dress that's quite becoming on Sarah herself — is not sympathy but fear. Daphne represents the terrible possibility, what she might be (or might have been) but probably (hopefully) isn't.

The problem for Sarah is the problem that troubled Charlotte Brontë and earlier women novelists — the problem of justice. If beauty is an arbitrary gift, like those other advantages, then it isn't fair that one woman should have it and another not. A chance encounter with Daphne at the Tate Gallery in London causes Sarah acute embarrassment. She herself is accompanied by a very well put-together male friend from Oxford. Daphne is alone, up for the weekend from the (presumably dismal) girls' school at which she teaches, and all too eager, it seems, to make the acquaintance of Sarah's friend. After they part and leave the gallery, Sarah's thoughts revert to Daphne. She wants so much to believe in life's infinite possibilities — not only (nor perhaps primarily) for Daphne, of

course, but for herself. Appearances, which seem to have everything to do with the air of failure Sarah sees in Daphne, *shouldn't*
matter. "Anyone can do anything," she affirms stoutly to her companion, as they stand on the steps of the gallery. "In theory perhaps," replies this impeccably dressed, successful, suave young
man. "I must say, it was a very curious color scheme." As they
wander the embankment along the river, the narrative perspective
is momentarily reversed. A little speedboat passes by, in which a
man and a girl in a headsquare are leaning against one another,
laughing: "You can do that, even on the greyest, dirtiest stretch of
river. It made me feel stagnant and covered in old and dead feathers,
to see them there." For a moment, Sarah sees herself as Daphne: *she*
is the one who stands alone, looking out at others' lives filled with
movement and intimacy, possibilities. And she reflects to herself:
"Daphne is somehow a threat to my existence. Whenever I see her,
I feel weighted down to earth. I feel the future narrowing before me
like a tunnel, and everyone else is high up and laughing" (chap. 7,
pp. 113–14).

Sarah keeps coming back to the problem of Daphne. In a later
scene, alone now in her dingy little London flat, she gets past the
superficial comparisons and comes to the heart of the problem: "I
do feel perpetually," she says, "the double-edged guilt and glory of
having so much, so much abundance: at school they tried to argue
it out of me by the 'Greater gifts — greater duties to society' line,
and I had swallowed it, at least as far as intellect went — but what
on earth was one to do about all this lovely body that one was
obliged to walk around with? . . . One can't shut one's eyes and
pretend it isn't so, or that, being so, it doesn't matter. It does matter. And yet," she continues, "there is no moral in it. I don't deserve
to be as I am: she doesn't deserve to be as she is. . . . Flesh is a
straight gift, I concluded" (chap. 10, pp. 167–68). Then, in what
seemed to me on my first reading and still seems to me now a wonderful gesture, complex in its awareness and honest in its celebration, Sarah, acting out a traditional ritual of heroines, looks at herself in her mirror. In performing that ritual, she does something her

pretty predecessors never do — or their creators never permitted them to do. Seeing herself staring back at herself, "caught in a paroxysm of vanity," "I hugged my own body in my own arms. My own flesh. Indisputable. Mine" (ibid.).

The specter of Daphne has haunted my life too — but in a way that is somewhat different from how Sarah is haunted. On the one hand, as a young woman, I identified more intensely than she with Daphne — with the unlucky, unprivileged, ugly woman. On the other hand, perhaps just because I have lived out that fate — and lived through it, I can better realize (*now* if not then) that Daphne's life has possibilities which Sarah, in her anxiety, cannot let herself see. If Sarah could let herself know Daphne better, she might discover why her cousin has, in Morrison's eloquent phrase "put on a cloak of ugliness" for the world. She might even be able to help her take it off, know herself as beautiful. At this stage in her own life, though, Sarah is too frightened to really see Daphne; she is too afraid of seeing in her the reflection of her own self — of a fate, if escaped, only narrowly and randomly so. Or, perhaps more precisely, Sarah is too afraid that between the smug self-absorption with which Louise attends to her body parts (there is a wonderful scene in which Louise forces the lover she has rejected to be the spectator of her elaborate grooming of her body) and the denial of the possibilities of the body Daphne emblemizes for her, there is no way for *her*. But there is a way.

And Sarah is acting it out in the very final moment of this scene. Though she calls it "a paroxysm of vanity," I would not call it that. Vanity is, as the word's Latin origins suggest, an emptiness — the real lack of self-love we see in the scene in which Louise combs her hair, in order to make a rejected suitor jealous, as she enters into a loveless marriage. There's a self-contempt, not real self-love, at the root of such vanity. But Sarah's action here, as she hugs her body in her own arms — "my own flesh. Indisputable. Mine" — is, as I read it, a healthy, self-affirming action, even as it contains the expression of her relief that she's *not* Daphne. She's delighting not only in having her own body, but in being her own self—a person who will ultimately be able to hug others in her own arms because she can hug herself in them. Maybe I liked Sarah, in my mid-twenties, not only because of the ways in which we were alike in our hopes and our anxieties, but because she had something I still needed—more of the basic love of herself in the body, more knowledge of herself as beautiful, lovable.

CHAPTER 4

Charlotte Brontë:
"As Small and as Plain as Myself"

*I*n the last chapter I described how, unconsciously at times and consciously at others, I have used my reading of fiction as a way of coming to terms with the beauty question in my own life. In the next two chapters I will discuss two great nineteenth-century women novelists who use their own writing of fiction for a similar purpose. Unlike the women novelists whose works we have been considering thus far (Burney, Austen, Gaskell, and Drabble), both Charlotte Brontë and George Eliot knew themselves as emphatically unattractive women; for each the beauty question was a personal and often a painful one. Those who recorded their first impressions on meeting each woman were quick to enumerate their respective defects in this category. To mention just a few, first, of Brontë: "She was at this time anything but pretty . . . all the plainer from her exceeding thinness and want of complexion, she looked 'dried in' ";[1] "a little, plain, provincial, sickly-looking old maid";[2] "Her head seemed too large for her body. She had fine eyes, but her face was marred by the shape of the mouth and by the complexion. There was but little feminine charm about her; and of this fact she was herself uneasily and perpetually conscious. . . . I believe she would have given all her genius and her fame to have been beautiful. Perhaps few women ever existed more anxious to be pretty than she, or more angrily conscious of the circumstance that she was not pretty."[3] And then of Eliot: "Her face is repulsively ugly from the immense size of the chin";[4] "Indeed one rarely sees a plainer woman; dull complexion, dull eyes, heavy features";[5] and, in the true patriarchal top-to-toe inventory-style: "To begin with, she is magnificently ugly — deliciously hideous. She has a low forehead, a dull grey eye, a vast pendulous nose, a huge mouth, full of uneven teeth, and a chin and jaw-bone *qui n'en finissent pas . . .*"[6] Only Brontë and Eliot themselves, as young women, were quicker than their observers to catalogue their physical flaws. Whether either was able to realize fully the process of becoming beautiful in her life is debatable; but each *was* emphatically, triumphantly, able to do so in her art, and thus to bequeath to us, in the body of her fiction, a model for the transformation of the ugly woman into the beautiful one — the "ugly" woman, I might better say, *realized* as the beautiful one.

It cannot be a coincidence that the two greatest women novelists of Victorian England were conspicuously lacking the conventional attributes of feminine beauty. Sir George White Pickering has written a fascinating book on the way illness (real or imagined) gave a number of great nineteenth- and early twentieth-century writers the freedom to concentrate more exclusively on what was the real business of their lives.[7] Chronic illness gave these men and women the freedom to reject a life in Victorian society, with all its myriad social as well as financial obligations, and to assume instead (without having to feel guilty) the life of essential solitude that was necessary if they were to pursue their true calling. In the same way, we might say that Brontë and Eliot consciously or unconsciously *chose* "ugliness," since a lack of conventional beauty freed them from the conventional Victorian woman's life — not a life in the world but rather one trapped within its interior confines. In an age when the number of marriageable women far exceeded that of marriageable men, and where marriage almost inevitably meant the subordination of the self to domestic life, these two "failures" were free to write (or Brontë was, at least, until her marriage with her father's curate, the Reverend Nicholls, in what was to be the final year of her life, when the writing ceased). More fully even than illness allows, the lack of conventional beauty in a woman gives her not only freedom *from* society but freedom to criticize its defects, since it has criticized hers. She may, specifically, show us in her fiction how a young woman who allows herself to be defined in the terms of the patriarchal beauty contest is preparing herself for a life in which her whole existence will be defined by others.

Elizabeth Gaskell, who was conventionally beautiful, happily married, and still wrote four great novels, might be seen as an exceptional woman novelist who managed somehow to have it all. But it is also true that, despite her daring exploration of such taboo issues as unwed motherhood, Gaskell, writing more securely from within her world, is a less intrepid chronicler of women's lives than either Brontë or Eliot. And for all its sympathy both for Brontë's life and her art, Elizabeth Gaskell's biography of her friend and fellow-novelist, Charlotte Brontë, remains basically an attempt to reclaim for Victorian respectability the woman whose frank exploration of female sexuality caused her novels to be labeled by many of her contemporaries as "coarse." It is not surprising that Brontë's oldest friend, Ellen Nussey, should have tried to secure a reproduction of the prettied-up Richmond portrait of Brontë for the Gaskell biography (a version of which graces the cover of my present Everyman paperback edition of that work as well as of my Penguin *Jane Eyre*), and that Ellen should have told Gaskell what a "satisfaction" it would be "to people to see something that would settle their ideas of the personal appearance of the dear departed one," adding, "it has been a surprise to every stranger, I think, that she was so gentle and lady-like to look upon."[8] So do the well-meaning impulses of our friends betray us both in life and in art. For neither in her avowed plainness nor in the difficult beauty she conferred on her heroines was Charlotte Brontë the "gentle and lady-like" figure of Richmond's portrait — the conventionally attractive, sweetly smiling woman whose image her friends wished to disseminate to the world. To portray her through such portraiture is to distort, subtly but emphatically, in the same way Gaskell's biography itself distorts, the radically subversive message of Brontë's art. But we may be in a better position today than were her contemporaries to value what Brontë has denied her heroine and what she affirms in her boast that she would give the world a heroine "as small and as plain as myself" who would still win the reader's sympathy.⁹ Her sisters doubted it could be done. But she did do it — defiantly, triumphantly.

Indeed, no one makes beauty, *seen as a mere appendage to the self,* seem more contemptible an advantage than Brontë does in *Jane Eyre.* From the very opening page of the novel, we see the orphaned child's heart saddened "by the chidings of Bessie, the nurse, and humbled by the consciousness of my physical inferiority to Eliza, John, and Georgiana Reed."¹⁰ And we see Jane's instinctive understanding that, "had I been a sanguine, brilliant, careless, exacting, handsome, romping child — though equally dependent and friendless — Mrs Reed would have endured my presence more complacently; her children would have entertained for me more of the cordiality of fellow-feeling; the servants would have been less prone to make me the scapegoat of the nursery" (chap. 2, p. 47). The cruel scapegoating of the ugly child, just because she *is* an ugly child, comes out clearly in this bit of dialogue between the two servants in the Reed household:

> Bessie, when she heard this narrative [of the death of Jane's parents], sighed and said, "Poor Miss Jane is to be pitied, too Abbot."
>
> "Yes," responded Abbot; "if she were a nice, pretty child, one might compassionate her forlornness; but one really cannot care for such a little toad as that."
>
> "Not a great deal, to be sure," agreed Bessie: "at any rate, a beauty like Miss Georgiana would be more moving in the same condition."
>
> "Yes, I dote on Miss Georgiana!" cried the fervent Abbot. "Little darling! — with her long curls and her blue eyes, and such a sweet colour as she has; just as if she were painted! — Bessie, I could fancy a Welsh rabbit for supper." *(chap. 3, p. 58)*

It is a radical moment in literary history. In defining the "compassion" traditionally elicited on behalf of pretty girls in distress as the sentiment of vulgar housemaids, Brontë exposes with one stroke of the pen the vulgarity that underlies centuries of romantic fiction. "Unjust! unjust!" we say, along with the young Jane Eyre: as a plain child she is all the *more* deserving of our compassion, because she is all the *more* deprived. Or as Brontë said to her sisters, when they doubted her plain heroine would win readers' hearts, it is wrong, "even *morally* wrong," for a writer to make her heroine beautiful, "as a matter of course."[11] In *Jane Eyre* Brontë makes us feel the immorality of the assumption that if she is to gain our compassion, a poor, forsaken little girl had better be sure she possesses beauty.

Whether they read her novel sympathetically or not, Brontë's early readers certainly got the point she was making with Jane's defiant plainness. They understood that her plainness, and not just her outspoken manner, constituted a repudiation of woman's supposed compliancy. Elizabeth Rigby, a writer, painter, and London socialite, wrote an essay on physiognomy for the *Quarterly Review* a few years after the publication of *Jane Eyre* in which she reminds her readers that "it is a woman's *business* to be beautiful."[12] In a review of *Jane Eyre* for the same periodical Rigby sees in the young Jane Eyre, "with her sharp eyes and dogmatic speeches . . . a being you neither could fondle nor love."[13] This description of Jane, along with Rigby's portrait, in the article on physiognomy, "of an unhappy anomalous style of young woman . . . who seems to have taken on herself the vows of voluntary ugliness — who neither eats enough to keep her complexion clear, nor smiles enough to set her pleasing muscles in action — who prides herself on a skinny parsimony of attire which she calls neatness — thinks that alone respectable which is most unbecoming — is always thin, and seldom well, and passes through the society of the lovely, the graceful, and the happy with the vanity that apes humility on her poor disappointed countenance; as if to say 'Stand back, I am uncomelier than thou . . .' " tells me that, on one level, Elizabeth Rigby understands Jane Eyre very well. She understands that the ugliness she sees in Jane and her real-life prototypes is, in the final analysis, a willed

ugliness, as much an act of hostility as it is one of self-effacement.
I agree with Rigby's statement that anyone *can* create a pleasing appearance in the world if they really wish to do so. She is insightful
enough to see the unhappiness and disappointment which hide beneath the facade of indifference to the world and its ways. Rigby
understands everything but the reason why a young woman might
well feel anguish at a destiny that demands it is her "business" to be
beautiful, a world which itself only smiles on a woman who is gen-
uinely happy to define herself in terms of the pleasure she provides
to others. Finally, Rigby's analysis is only a more sophisticated version of Bessie and Abbot's preference for the "darling" (accom-
modating) Georgiana.

The economist and literary critic Walter Bagehot got the point
of Jane's plainness too — and saw its import from the perspective
of a male reader, or purveyor. In an 1858 essay, lamenting the dis-
appearance from the contemporary literary scene of the ideally
beautiful, compliant heroine of Scott's fiction, Bagehot observes in
passing that "possibly none of the frauds which are now so much
the topic of common remark are so irritating, as that to which the
purchaser of a novel is a victim on finding that he has only to peruse
a narrative of the conduct and sentiments of an ugly lady."[14] The
male purchaser of *Jane Eyre*, in the three-volume edition which was
standard for the time, has laid out a fair sum — not only for the
book but (implicitly) for the woman who is its heroine; and he has
not got his money's worth! Never mind that Bagehot's comment is
meant to amuse: it takes my breath away. And yet it is only a cruder
version of what Jane's own lover, Rochester, says to Jane when he
tells her, "I will myself put the diamond chain around your
neck, . . . and I will clasp the bracelets on these fine wrists, and load
these fairy-like fingers with rings" (all these, family heirlooms he
has ordered his banker to send from London) and "will make the
world acknowledge you a beauty, too" (chap. 24, pp. 287, 288).
Jane's anguished protest — "Don't address me as if I were a beauty;
I am your plain, Quakerish governess" (chap. 24, p. 287) — comes
from deep in her heart. Her lover's language here, with its sugges-

tion not only of enslavement but of turning the small, slight woman into a heavy one, loaded down with the weight of her future husband's family's jewels, is a vivid metaphor for the threatened submergence of Jane's identity in his. But Rochester is paying his attentions to Jane in the only language he has learned to speak to women, which is that of prostitution — the language of Bagehot's talk about his fraudulent purchase and (at bottom) of Rigby's talk about women's "business" as well. So Jane rightly categorizes such beauty talk when she says to Rochester later, "Do you remember what you said of [his French mistress] Céline Varens? — of the diamonds, the cashmeres you gave her? I will not be your English Céline Varens" (chap. 24, p. 298). But Rochester needs time to learn a different kind of language with which to make love to Jane; and his education is also our education.

There is a rightness, then, in the fact that, at the critical point of proposing marriage to her, Rochester does not err but appropriates Jane's own terminology for herself, saying, "You — poor and obscure, and small and plain as you are — I entreat to accept me as a husband" (chap. 23, p. 283). Rochester is, to be sure, teasing Jane a bit here by echoing the epithets she herself used earlier in this same conversation, when he was dilating on the attractions of his supposed bride-to-be, the beautiful Blanche Ingram. Jane responded to this cruel test by declaring herself, as he hoped she would, in no uncertain terms: "Do you think, because I am poor, obscure, plain, and little, I am soulless and heartless?" (p. 281). Her way of seeing herself is not necessarily his way. Yet there is a fitness in his appropriation of the terms she has so recently used to describe herself, as he tells her it is she, not the beautiful Blanche, he really loves. For in choosing a "small" woman he is, symbolically, choosing one who will not allow her body to be encumbered by the Rochester family jewels or by the weight of custom and conventionalities that go with them. And in choosing the "plain" woman he is choosing a woman who will not allow her person to be used to raise her husband's account in the eyes of the world. "Plain" in the first half of the nineteenth century, let us also remember, had not yet come to be simply the euphemism for "ugly" it is today; the term still has strong associations of freedom — with honest "plain" dealings, with unadorned "plain" dress, and with unaffected "plain" speech.

And yet, at the same time, no one makes beauty, seen not as an appendage to the self but *as an expression of the self,* seem more precious than Brontë does in *Jane Eyre.* To understand the preciousness of the beauty she confers on Jane Eyre, I think we have to explore more fully the etiology of Brontë's sense of her own plainness — more particularly, of her plainness-as-smallness, for the two terms in her parlance are always joined. Why should smallness have been, at least in the beginning, the very definition of her unattractiveness? Extremely small Charlotte Brontë undoubtedly was, the smallest woman in a family of small women — four foot nine inches, according to the joiner who made her coffin,[15] which is unusually small even for the early nineteenth century. Yet smallness, particularly in that era, was not viewed as undesirable in a woman. But the terms Brontë uses in speaking to Gaskell about her smallness provide a clue: she describes herself as "stunted"[16] and "underdeveloped"[17] — terms Gaskell herself emphatically rejects.[18] Brontë's own analysis of the cause of her "stuntedness" takes us a step further: "Her stunted person she ascribed to a scanty supply of food she had as a growing girl, when at that school of the Daughters of the Clergy." Harriet Martineau elaborates: "She was never free while there . . . from the gnawing sensation or consequent feebleness of downright hunger; and she never grew an inch from that time. She was the smallest of women; and it was that school which stunted her growth."[19] Her smallness — at least in Brontë's own mind, if not necessarily in fact — is associated with a lack of essential nurture in her formative childhood years. In *Jane Eyre* Brontë suggests a similar explanation for her heroine's smallness. Her old nurse Bessie, seeing Jane after her eight years at Lowood (under which name Brontë makes infamous the school she and her two elder sisters attended for a year with such grievous results) comments: "You're not grown so very tall, Miss Jane, nor so very stout . . . I dare say they've not kept you too well at school, Miss Reed is the head and shoulders taller than you are; and Miss Georgiana would make two of you in breadth" (chap. 10, p. 122).[20] The truth about the quality of the food at the Cowan's Bridge school and whether an inadequate diet could have had such a "stunting" effect on the growth of a child who remained there for such a short period are debatable issues.[21] But it is undeniable that at Cowan Bridge Charlotte was very unhappy; it is the place where two beloved elder sisters died in a typhus epidemic. She could easily have felt severely malnourished there, on a psychological level.

I suspect some of the anger Brontë directs toward the institution where she spent her eighth year has its source in deprivations experienced at home in the several years immediately preceding her year at Cowan Bridge. When Charlotte was four her father moved his family from the town of Thornton, where he and his wife had enjoyed a large circle of friends and cultural activities, to the isolated parsonage in the tiny village of Haworth. Then, a few months later, following the birth of the fifth and last child, Mrs. Brontë became ill with cancer, and (to quote a recent biographer) "spent the next seven months dying in the hushed atmosphere of the little house, so ill that Mr Brontë expected her death almost every day. It was a terrifying long-drawn-out experience for the children, whose father was too impatient and distraught to be of comfort. . . . [After his wife's death he] did not suffer his loss stoically, and seems to have found his children's presence a painful reminder of his wife rather than a comfort. . . . The gay, gregarious side of his nature slowly became submerged; he withdrew into himself, beginning the habit of dining alone, theoretically on account of his poor digestion."[22] The fact of her father's withdrawal from his children after their mother's death and particularly his absenting himself from the literal and symbolic center of their place of nourishment — the family dinner table — may help us better understand Charlotte's own life-long association between her smallness and her plainness. Her later explanation for her "stunted person" would seem an unconscious expression of anger and grief, not only for her mother's death but for the subsequent withdrawal of her father's love.

In her early years, and indeed throughout her life, Brontë connects her sense of her "stunted person" with a fear that she may not be seen at all. It is the same link between a sense of the self as unsightly and the sense of the self as invisible that we saw in Burney's Eugenia. But Brontë continually courts the feared invisibility — as the small woman makes herself even smaller by "shrinking" from sight. So does Ellen Nussey, who was to become Charlotte's lifelong friend, describe her first sight of Charlotte at the age of fourteen as a new pupil at the Roe Head School. Ellen, herself a new arrival, was standing, as she thought, alone in the schoolroom —

> when, turning to the window to observe the look-out I became aware for the first time that I was not alone; there was a silent, weeping, dark little figure in the large bay-window; she must, I thought, have risen from the floor. As soon as I had recovered from my surprise, I went from the far end of the room, where the bookshelves were, the contents of which I must have contemplated with a little awe in anticipation of coming studies. A crimson cloth covered the long table down the centre of the room, which helped no doubt to hide the shrinking little figure from my view. I was touched and troubled at once to see her so sad and tearful.[23]

It is not surprising that a new girl on the first day of school should be sad and tearful. But the contrast between the body language of the two new girls here is striking: Ellen first looks at the books, thinking ahead to the coming school year, albeit with some trepidation; Charlotte hides, perhaps at first on the floor but then in the setting occupied by all her heroines, the window seat. There she may or may not be seen, and can herself observe the activity of the persons in the room — but from a safe vantage point. Ellen takes the initiative, moving toward the "little figure" whom she has seen, thus taking the first step in what would become a lifelong friendship; while, Charlotte, by contrast, "shrinks" — the small person literally making herself even smaller. Ellen comments: "I said shrinking because her attitude, when I saw her, was that of one who wished to hide both herself and her grief."[24] The "shrinking" person *is* hiding both herself and her grief — her grief at being insufficiently cherished. And she is at the same time insisting that, if there is to be a meeting, the other person must be the one to initiate it, to discover the "small and plain" person shrinking in her corner and let her know she is noticed, is cared for — as Ellen does in this encounter. There is a corresponding sense of Charlotte having to be coaxed into eating at Roe Head (where presumably there was no defect in the food itself). Ellen comments: "Her appetite was of the smallest; for years she had not tasted animal food; she had the greatest dislike to it; she always had something specially provided for her at our midday repast. Toward the close of the first half-year she was induced to take, by little and little, meat gravy with vegetable, and in the second half-year she commenced taking a very small portion of animal food daily. She then grew a little plumper, looked younger and more animated, though she was never what is called lively at this period."[25] The connection between the animal food Charlotte refuses and the animal spirits Ellen sees lacking in her (a connection which operates both on a linguistic and a psychological level) suggests to me a very deep-seated response to the early denial of affection from the animate world — the world that can and should provide nourishment for a child.

Brontë staged all of her future meetings with strangers as a test of the other's love, parallel to that first meeting with Ellen Nussey. Gaskell describes the young Charlotte in Brussels who had a habit "before her tongue was loosened . . . of gradually wheeling round on her chair so as almost to conceal her face from the person to whom she was speaking,"[26] as well as her encounter with the writer in later years as "a little lady in a black silk gown, whom I could not see at first for the dazzle of the room . . . [who] work[ed] away and hardly spoke."[27] Gaskell also connects Brontë's shrinking manner with her anxiety about her own plainness — her feeling that others will not want to look at her.

> Much of [her] nervous dread of encountering strangers I ascribed to the idea of her personal ugliness, which had been strongly impressed upon her imagination early in life, and which she exaggerated to herself in a remarkable manner. "I notice," said she, "that after a stranger has once looked at my face, he is careful not to let

his eyes wander to that part of the room again!" A more untrue idea never entered into any one's head. Two gentlemen who saw her during this visit [in the spring of 1853, after her fame as the author of *Jane Eyre* as well as of *Shirley* and *Villette* was established], without knowing at the time who she was, were singularly attracted by her appearance; and this feeling of attraction toward a pleasant countenance, sweet voice, and gentle timid manners, was so strong in one as to conquer a dislike he had previously entertained to her works.[28]

In Gaskell's own portrait of Brontë in the biography we can see the lineaments of the "difficult" beauty we have seen before in nineteenth-century women's fiction. She may "pretty up" Brontë's image for us on a moral level, but Gaskell saw the beauty of "countenance" in Brontë's person; and she gives it to us in a wonderful portrait that focuses particularly on her friend's "peculiar eyes, of which I find it difficult to give a description, as they appeared to me in her later life. They were large, and well shaped; their colour a reddish brown; but if the iris was closely examined, it appeared to be composed of a great variety of tints. The usual expression was of quiet, listening intelligence; but now and then, on some just occasion for vivid interest or wholesome indignation, a light would shine out, as if some spiritual lamp had been kindled, which glowed behind those expressive orbs. I never saw the like in any other human creature." As for the rest of her features, "they were plain, large, and ill set; but, unless you began to catalogue them" — which is just what she will not do — "you were hardly aware of the fact, for the eyes and power of the countenance overbalanced every physical defect; the crooked mouth and the large nose were forgotten, and the whole face arrested the attention, and presently attracted all those whom she herself would have cared to attract."[29]

There it all is: the very beauty that Brontë does confer on her "small and plain" heroines, but sadly, it would seem, was never able to recognize in herself. Her curious comment here that a stranger, having looked in her direction is careful *not* to let his eye wander to that part of the room again might be read as a statement of the intensity of her desire that he do so. Again and again, narratives of first meetings with Charlotte Brontë are structured around the issue of recognition: will the Currer Bell incognito — under which *Jane Eyre* was published and which Brontë insisted not be unmasked for as long as two years after that novel and the identity of its mysterious author had been the talk of London — be uncovered? Will the plain and small woman sitting silently in the corner be recognized as Charlotte Brontë the great author? But beneath the question of the discovery of the identity of the literary celebrity there is always the deeper question: will the shrinking little woman be seen — and loved — at all?

In her mature art, if not in her life, Brontë was able to effect the transformation of the "small and plain" woman into the beautiful woman — even as she *remains*, as we have already seen in *Jane Eyre*, defiantly, triumphantly, small and plain. But at the very start of her fictional career, in the early juvenilia and unpublished novelettes, the beautiful woman who assumes the center of the stage is precisely her own antitype. Her portraits of these heroines suggest she felt that a woman could be seen and loved only by assuming that posture which she herself could not and would not ever assume — by literally "imposing" herself upon the viewer. Thus of Zenobia Ellvington, in the unpublished 1834 narrative, "A Peep into a Picture-Book," the narrator exclaims: "What eyes! What raven hair! What an imposing contour of form and countenance. She is perfectly grand in her velvet robes, dark plume and crown-like turban."[30] And, a few years later, of the heroine of *Julia*: " 'Magnificent contour!' repeated Warner impatiently, and . . . pointed to an open window, where, suffused by the glow of crimson hangings drawn before the sunlight, sat a fine woman of about nine and twenty. She was dark in complexion, not very tall, but in all her forms round and superb . . . "[31] And, a year later, in 1839, the heroine of *Mina Laury* is seen crossing "the large light passage, such an apparition of feminine elegance and beauty — she had dressed herself splendidly — the robe of black satin became at once her slender form, which it enveloped in full & shining folds . . . "[32]

These are large, grand women, their size made all the more conspicuous by their voluminous clothing — women seen and admired
as they move through realms of light. In such company the small
"shrinking" woman is apt to be, literally, unseen. "Oh! I had forgotten to introduce you to my cousin, Marian," says a character in
Brontë's first attempt at a full-scale novel, *Ashworth* (1840–41). "I
beg pardon but she is so tiny, it is easy to overlook her."[33]

We might neatly locate the beginning of Brontë's mature fiction
at the point where the spectator ceases to turn away from the "small
and plain" woman and turns instead *toward* her, seeking her out in
her dark corner — or in other words, at the point where the woman
novelist allows herself to love — and thus invites her reader to
love — a heroine who is an extension of rather than an opposite to
her own physical self. The emergence of Brontë as a great novelist
thus coincides with her placing herself — as a loved figure — at the
center of her fiction. But it takes time: the full realization of the
small and plain heroine as a beautiful woman (in the eyes of those
who know and love her) comes only with *Jane Eyre*. We may
glimpse the beginning of this transforming vision, however, in the
portrait of Elizabeth Hastings, the heroine of *Captain Henry Hastings* (1839), the last of the juvenilian novelettes, who is first seen in
the grey, uncertain light of dawn, an unknown "shrinking" figure
wrapped in a shawl. "Being but little and thin," the masculine narrator comments, "she was easily stowed away between myself and
a stout woman in a plurality of cloaks."[34] That stout woman has no
part to play in the ensuing narrative: but she is there that we may
see the emergence of the small and plain heroine as an act of usurpation! For the stout woman is the grand beauty of the early
fiction — with all her imposing grandeur converted into lumpish
(intrusive) weight and her gorgeous attire into an excess of wraps.
So later we are told that "had [Elizabeth] dressed herself stylishly
and curled her hair, no one would have called her plain — but in a
brown silk frock — a simple collar and hair parted on her forehead
in smooth braids — she was just an insignificant — unattractive
young woman wholly without the bloom — majesty or fullness of

beauty."[35] But "bloom," "majesty," and "fullness" are losing their status in Brontë's fiction as the indices of beauty.

In *The Professor*, Brontë's first novel, written in 1846, a year before *Jane Eyre* but not published until after her death, in 1857, the "small and plain" woman moves a step closer, sexually speaking, to the center of the stage. That she does so is linked to a decisive event in Brontë's own life — her sojourn in Brussels, between 1842 and 1844, as a teacher of English and a student of French. It was in the Belgian Pensionnat of Mme. Heger that Charlotte fell passionately in love with the husband of the school's mistress, M. Heger — himself a brilliant and dynamic teacher, who was to become the model for Rochester in *Jane Eyre* and for M. Paul Emanuel in Brontë's last novel, *Villette*. Though her feeling for M. Heger was unreciprocated and probably not recognized for what it was at the time even by Charlotte herself, the intense emotions awakened by what was to be the decisive romantic attachment of her life surely helped turn the focus of sexual attention in her fiction to a woman who is her prototype rather than her antitype. In the preface she wrote for an anticipated publication of *The Professor* in 1851, Brontë declares that she "had got over any such taste as I might once have had for ornamented and redundant composition, and come to prefer was was plain and homely,"[36] signalling at once a change in prose style and in heroine style. Notice how Brontë invites us to see her heroine by having her narrator the schoolmaster (the masculine figure is still assuming the narrator's role) correct his own way of seeing her.

> I had been accustomed to nurse a flattering idea that my strong attachment to her proved some particular perspicacity in my nature; she was not handsome, she was not rich, she was not even accomplished, yet she was my life's treasure; I must then be a man of peculiar discernment. Tonight my eyes opened on the mistake I had made. . . . It is true Frances' mental points had been the first to interest me, and they still retained the strongest hold on my preference; but I liked the graces of her person too. I derived a pleasure, purely material, from contemplating the clearness of her brown

eyes, the fairness of her fine skin, the purity of her well-set teeth,
the proportion of her delicate form; and that pleasure I could ill
have dispensed with. It appeared, then, that I too was a sensualist,
in my temperate and fastidious way.   *(chap. 23, p. 188)*

We may imagine that Brontë herself came in for a certain amount
of this sort of "flattering" talk from the several earnest suitors she
rejected as a young woman, and perhaps from those men she did
not have the opportunity to reject! In *The Professor* she gives her
masculine protagonist the chance to correct himself, to make clear
that he loves Frances Henri not just for her mental beauty but for
her physical charm.

Compared to Jane Eyre's, the "difficult" beauty of Frances
Henri is easy. Frances Henri may be no striking beauty, but her regular features, right proportions, and well-set teeth, are all duly
noted. With Frances Henri Brontë still fudges the size issue somewhat: when the narrator first sees her with the eyes of love he no-
tices a change in her person: "her figure . . . became rounder, and
as the harmony of her form was complete and her stature of the
graceful middle height, one did not regret (or at least *I* did not regret) the absence of confirmed fulness . . . " (chap. 18, p. 120).
Gaskell, significantly, wanted to see *The Professor* published after
Brontë's death, in part because she thought it contained "the most
charming woman she ever drew."[37] But the beauty of Jane Eyre
makes no such compromises; there are no concessions to the re-
quirements of the classical canon. And if Jane's beauty is less obvious, her lover's passion is all the more overt: there is nothing
fastidious or temperate in Rochester's sexual feeling for Jane. In
no other mid-nineteenth-century novel is a heroine's "difficult"
beauty more "difficult" than in *Jane Eyre*. And, at the same time, in
no other novel of the period does an author make such a claim on
her heroine's behalf — both as the object of a deep sexual passion
and as one who feels such passion herself. The radicalness of *Jane
Eyre* might be described in terms of the tension it maintains between its presentation of a heroine who is at once plain *and* emphatically desirable.

When Jane insists that Rochester not address her as a beauty, he demurs; but even as he continues to speak in the old terms, he is beginning to learn (from her) a new beauty language: "You are a beauty in my eyes, and a beauty just after the desire of my heart — delicate and aerial (chap. 24, p. 288). Seen thus, with the eyes of love, Jane's smallness becomes associated not with deprivation but with the dearness of something easily lost — as when, in other passages, Rochester terms her his "elusive elf," "a pale little elf," and "a mustard-seed." If only Jane had been able to attend to the words in which Rochester delivers his feigned praise of Blanche Ingram's beauty! If only she had listened when he says, "She's an extensive armful: but that's not to the point — one can't have too much of such a very excellent thing as my beautiful Blanche" (chap. 23, p. 279), would she not have heard him telling her whom he *really* thinks is beautiful, whom he *really* loves? Of course she would have! Because all through *Jane Eyre*, the narrative voice, the voice of Brontë's mature fiction, is telling us very clearly how to see beauty — as the extension of its creator's own person. And, familiar as we are with that voice by this point in the narrative, we know that the woman who demands that her weight be borne by another (no fairy elf she, no mustard seed) is not a beautiful woman, not someone upon whom this narrator bestows her own loving gaze.

The scene where Jane prepares her toilette to go downstairs on the first morning of her new life as a governess at Thornfield, where (though she does not yet know it) a sexual passion will soon be awakened in her, deserves a careful reading. If we are willing to read between the lines of her reflexive self-deprecation on the subject, we may discover a new note of confidence in Jane about her life in her own body:

> I rose; I dressed myself with care: obliged to be plain — for I had no article of attire that was not made with extreme simplicity — I was still by nature solicitous to be neat. It was not my habit to be disregardful of appearance, or careless of the impression I made; on the contrary, I ever wished to look as well as I could, and to please as much as my want of beauty would permit. I sometimes regretted

that I was not handsomer: I sometimes wished to have rosy cheeks, a straight nose, and small cherry mouth: I desired to be tall, stately, and finely developed in figure; I felt it a misfortune that I was so little, so pale, and had features so irregular and so marked. And why had I these aspirations and these regrets? It would be difficult to say: I could not then distinctly say it to myself; yet I had a reason, and a logical, natural reason too. However, when I had brushed my hair very smooth, and put on my black frock — which Quaker-like as it was, at least had the merit of fitting to a nicety — and adjusted my clean white tucker, I thought I should do respectably enough to appear before Mrs Fairfax; and that my new pupil would not at least recoil from me with antipathy. Having opened my chamber window, and seen that I had left all things straight and neat on the toilet-table, I ventured forth.   *(chap. 11, p. 130)*

Some readers may feel only the tentativeness, the hesitation here, and perhaps prudishness rather than any blossoming sensuality in Jane's comments about her neat, orderly person in its well-fitting Quakerish dress. But I see Jane beginning to define herself as a sexual person in her own terms: the Quakerish dress, that has the advantage of fitting "to a nicety," is, after all, a dress that reveals the contours of the body within it. And while the passage acknowledges the regret she sometimes feels at not conforming to the world's image of the ideally beautiful woman, we may notice that the particular elements of beauty Jane isolates here — those of a woman whose features (all but that "small cherry mouth") imply largeness and grandeur — define only one style of beauty. What I like particularly in this passage is the way it registers the complexity of Jane's feelings at a moment of turning. For as she turns to descend the stairs, she is at a turning point in her life; and her feelings express both a wish for a style of beauty she could feel confident would meet general acceptance and a hope for something better than that — that as she takes care of her body herself, it may be loved for itself, as it is. Important too is Jane's understanding (now if not then) that she has a good reason for "these aspirations and these regrets": she is beginning to see the vital connection between an affirmation of her life in the body and her knowledge of herself as a person who is loving and capable of being loved.

On the morning when she dresses herself after Rochester's proposal of marriage, Jane is ready for a considerably larger assertion:

> While arranging my hair, I looked at my face in the glass, and felt it was no longer plain: there was hope in its aspect and life in its colour; and my eyes seemed as if they had beheld the fount of fruition, and borrowed beams from the lustrous ripple. I had often been unwilling to look at my master, because I feared he could not be pleased at my look: but I was sure I might lift my face to his now, and not cool his affection by its expression. I took a plain but clean and light summer dress from my drawer and put it on: it seemed no attire had ever so well become me, because none had I ever worn in so blissful a mood. *(chap. 24, p. 286)*

As her assumption of a "plain but clean and light dress" may remind us, what Jane sees in her mirror is not a changed image of her body, but the image of herself in love — which is what Rochester sees too, when he greets her: " 'Jane, you look blooming, and smiling, and pretty,' said he: 'truly pretty this morning. Is this my pale little elf? Is this my mustard-seed? This sunny-faced girl with the dimpled cheek and rosy lips; the satin-smooth hazel hair, and the radiant hazel eyes?' (I had green eyes, reader; but you must excuse the mistake; for him they were new-dyed, I suppose.)" (ibid., p. 287). Yes, new-dyed, *for both of them.* So in this part-real and part-illusory period of courtship, and then, more fully still, in the delayed marriage which finally perfects it (after all the complications of the other Mrs. Rochester have been resolved), Jane is known by both of them as at once the "small and plain Quakerish governess" *and* as a beautiful woman. There is no contradiction here, no "fairy tale" have-your-cake-and-eat-it-too; for both affirmations have, at bottom, the same source: Jane's rejection of all that is false to her true self.

It is ironic that Brontë should often be remembered as a writer who would have us honor moral rather than physical beauty. For a respect for her "moral beauty" is precisely what the self-righteous

St. John Rivers offers Jane — and what she decisively rejects. To the minister she is, from first to last, physically unattractive: "Ill or well, she would always be plain. The grace and harmony of beauty are quite wanting in those features" (chap. 29, p. 366). St. John reserves his sexual passion for another woman, and in proposing to Jane declares her "formed for labour, not for love" (chap. 34, p. 428). His proposal sums up a way of looking at herself that Jane has been struggling with ever since her early days at Gateshead (as a supremely useful rather than an intrinsically lovable human being) and is now ready to reject, as she turns, in ecstatic flight, back to Rochester.

Bertha's fortuitous death, of course, makes a marriage possible; but before she knows of the fire and its consequences, Jane knows she will spend the rest of her life close to this man who felt for her what no one ever did before, and who saw her as no one ever did or would see her again: "The servants say they never saw anybody so much in love as he was: he was after her continually. They used to watch him — servants will, you know, ma'am — and he set store on her past everything: for all, nobody but him thought her so very handsome. She was a little, small thing, they say, almost like a child . . . " (chap. 36, pp. 451–52). It's not vanity that sends Jane running back to Rochester — the vanity of a woman who thinks, "he loves me and finds me attractive even if no one else does." It's her knowledge that Rochester is the one man who really knows her, and seeing her as she is sees her as beautiful. (Her new-found cousins, Diana and Mary, who also know and love Jane, see her beauty too.)[38]

Jane Eyre broke new ground through Brontë's insistence that her plain heroine could become the object of love and desire, and also by portraying sexual seeing and discovery as reciprocal. As Rochester discovers her beauty, Jane's discovery of his beauty is a way for her to discover and claim her own sexual feelings. The man in whom she initially sees no beauty (and feels comfortable with on that account — no sexual tensions to worry about),[39] she discovers to be beautiful, as she discovers she loves him: "And was Mr Rochester now ugly in my eyes?" and answers: "No, reader: gratitude and many associations, all pleasurable and genial, made his face the object I best liked to see; his presence in a room was more cheering than the brightest fire" (chap. 15, p. 178). The same revisionary seeing is at the same time taking place in him — though she does not yet know it. And her changed perception of him is heightened, just as his is of her, by the failure of the world to see what each sees in the other. The drawing Jane makes of the beloved face on her return visit to Gateshead, feeling well pleased with her rendition of the broad forehead, square jaw, and strongly marked features, is pronounced by the undiscerning (and of course, no longer pretty-as-a-picture) Georgiana to be the face of "an ugly man" (chap. 21, pp. 261, 62). Once we allow that the pleasure we take in the physical aspect of a loved person is linked to the pleasure we take in getting to know that person, then it becomes possible to allow that women as well as men have sexual desires.

In *Jane Eyre* Brontë achieves a wonderful balance between the small and plain — but free — heroine and the beautiful, loved heroine. It is, as it must be, a precarious balance for one who has a strong need for autonomy and an equally strong need for union and the submergence of the self in mature sexual love. It is not surprising that in her last novel, *Villette*, the balance is not consistently sustained. Published six years later (in 1853), Brontë's darkest novel (*Shirley* was published between the two, in 1849) was written after the deaths of both her beloved sisters, Emily and Anne, as well as that of the sadly degenerated Branwell, and after the death of any lingering hope she may have had that a Rochester would enter her own life. In *Jane Eyre* the revenge Brontë takes against her antitype — the large, imposingly beautiful woman — still tastes sweet. We can feel glee when Jane, flushed with the new self-confidence she has gained at Thornfield and beginning to know her importance to Rochester, returns to the scene of her childhood humiliations, sees again her first rival Georgiana, and sees "not the Georgiana I remembered — the slim and fairy-like girl of eleven," but "a full-blown, very plump damsel, fair as wax work, with

handsome and regular features, languishing blue eyes, and ring-
leted yellow hair" (chap. 21, p. 257). In *Villette* the distaste Brontë
expresses for women who are such "extensive armfuls" seems more
like disgust than gratified revenge — and perhaps like something
else, fear. *Villette* is a reworking of the Brussels experience and
Brontë's passion for M. Heger, but told this time from the woman's
point of view, and with all the agony of that passion and the confused turmoil of her feelings exposed. Though the heroine, Lucy
Snowe, is loved and found beautiful by her schoolmaster-lover at
the novel's end, we are not allowed to hope for a permanent union
between these lovers; and, compared to *Jane Eyre*, the whole novel
speaks more intensely of passion's frustration than its gratification.
On the one hand, Lucy Snowe has more intense sexual longings
than Jane Eyre — or her longings are more evident on the surface of
the narrative. And on the other hand, there is a strong sense that her
longings will never be satisfied. This heroine's frustration and anger
at a passion that must be thwarted and repressed are linked to the
deeper distaste she expresses for her rival — the large, conspicuously beautiful woman. One feels it in a passage where Lucy
Snowe, a schoolmistress, is taking her pupils out for a walk. One
of the pupils, the comely and much-presuming Ginevra Fanshawe,
has attracted the man to whom Lucy herself is initially drawn. As
they walk, Ginevra leans upon Lucy's arm, forcing her to support
"the dear pressure of that angel's not unsubstantial limb."[40] And
Lucy adds, with an exaggeration of the facetious tone of Rochester's encomium to Blanche, that "many a time in the course of that
warm day I wished to goodness there had been less of that charming commodity" (chap. 33, p. 470). Here the "extensive armful"
acts out in literal terms the very thing the small heroine consistently
refuses to do: she demands to be supported. A part of Lucy's distaste here surely comes from the small and free woman's lingering
fear of being engulfed, taken over, by the larger, more compelling
person. But perhaps Ginevra also seems revolting to Lucy Snowe
because, in demanding to be supported, she is doing something a
Brontë heroine could never permit herself to do.

There are moments in *Villette* when one wonders whether sexuality itself, at once desired and despaired of, becomes the focus for Lucy's anger. I ask myself that question particularly when reading a remarkable scene in which Lucy tours the picture-gallery in Villette and sees a painting that is evidently "the queen of the collection," a huge tableau of the naked Cleopatra, before which is placed a bench for the accommodation of worshipping connoisseurs. Lucy's cold, clinical eye registers the fact that this Cleopatra

> was, indeed, extremely well fed: very much butcher's meat — to say nothing of bread, vegetables, and liquids — must she have consumed to attain that breadth and height, that wealth of muscle, that affluence of flesh. She lay half-reclined on a couch: why, it would be difficult to say; broad daylight blazed round her; she appeared in hearty health, strong enough to do the work of two plain cooks; she could not plead a weak spine; she ought to have been standing, or at least sitting bolt upright. She had no business to lounge away the noon on a sofa. She ought likewise to have worn decent garments; a gown covering her properly, which was not the case: out of abundance of material — seven-and-twenty yards, I should say, of drapery — she managed to make inefficient raiment. Then, for the wretched untidiness surrounding her, there could be no excuse. *(chap. 19, pp. 275–76)*

Part of this heroine's contempt for such an icon is that of the free Protestant in the alien Catholic world of idolatry and superstition. But Lucy's voice also has in it something of the tone of a young child whose protests about what the grown-ups are doing in bed covers some real distress at what is seen but only partly understood. In all this disorderly profusion of flesh and drapery and "pots and pans," is sex itself the real enemy? I think in Brontë, and particularly in *Villette*, there is a real anxiety about the blurring of boundaries which is an inevitable part of the sexual encounter. The precarious balance *Jane Eyre* celebrates, a balance so crucial to Brontë in her own life, is lost in *Villette* — as indeed it so often is in life.

But if *Villette* as a whole fails to reconcile Brontë's own desire for passionate self-surrender with her equally strong desire for autonomy, there is an image in this novel, and in her fiction generally, for such a union. All those neat little houses in Brontë's fiction, which fit her heroines as nicely as their clothing always fits their bodies, and are tended by them with as much care, have a strong sexual charge — the positive pole to the negative sexual charge of Cleopatra's messy domain. In a recurrent scene in Brontë's fiction the chosen male enters the heroine's tiny, immaculate "nutshell" of a house and sees with delighted eyes the world she has made within. It is the world of the small and plain, where everything is in its proper place, everything "suits," and all is lovingly cared for. The first version of this house is Frances Henri's small apartment in *The Professor*, seen here, with its mistress inside it, as Crimsworth visits her home for the first time, and "stepping over a little mat of green wool," finds himself in a small room, whose articles of furniture are few "but all bright and exquisitely clean." In the entrance to this little home, which we can see as a metaphor for the man's delighted gaze and discovery of the woman's inner, sexual parts, "order reigns through its narrow limits." As an image for paradise, this is the Renaissance poet George Herbert's "box where sweets compacted lie" rather than John Milton's "enormous bliss." But it is a sexual paradise all the same. And Frances's own emergence, as she returns to the front room, having taken off her bonnet, to make her guest at home, reinforces that sense, for she comes out, "a model of frugal neatness, with her well-fitting black stuff dress, so accurately defining her elegant bust and taper waist, with her spotless white collar turned back from a fair and shapely neck. . . . Ornaments she had none — neither brooch, ring, nor ribbon; she did well enough without them — perfection of fit, proportion of form, grace of carriage, agreeably supplied their place" (chap. 19, p. 141). Sartorially speaking, the well-fitting garment we see here on Frances Henri is the emblem of the Brontë heroine. As always with clothing, what counts is less the particular cut and style of the garment than the look and feel of the clothing on the body. And in the Frances Henri passage it is particularly evident that the sort of dress we might be tempted to denigrate today as a robe of constriction is, for this wearer at least, one that expresses or "defines" not just the shape of the body but the quality of the person within it.

The equivalent house in *Jane Eyre* is a gayer and a more inclusive home, as befits Brontë's most expansive novel. Moor House is never Jane's very own house; nor is it conferred on her by her lover. But at a critical state in her development Moor House takes on important symbolic overtones as an emblem of her new self-assurance, and particularly of her sexual self-assurance. Jane discovers that she is not the friendless and moneyless orphan she had thought she was, but is cousin to the two women she has come to love and know as her true soul-mates. As the heir to her uncle's large estate, she can redeem her cousins from their planned lives of joyless toil as governesses among strangers. They can all come home, and the home, as the money, will be shared equally among them all. The first thing Jane does with her new wealth — and, symbolically, it is a highly important action — is thoroughly to clean and redecorate Moor House. For she is, in the act, which is also a communal act of love, preparing her own body to receive Rochester. Moor House is a "pretty little" house to begin with, "exquisitely neat," and Jane will not alter it — any more than she will deck her own person out in Rochester's family heirlooms. But she throws herself into the action of cleaning, and polishing, and perfecting the little dwelling with a joyous energy we have not seen in her till now. Hannah, the maid, is "charmed to see how jovial I could be amidst the bustle of a house turned topsy-turvy — how I could dust, and brush, and clean, and cook. And really," Jane continues, "after a day or two of confusion worse confounded, it was delightful by degrees to invoke order from the chaos ourselves had made" (chap. 34, p. 417). There is a nice sense here, if we read the scene symbolically, of the heroine as the caretaker of her own body, her own beauty — which is linked to the pleasure she feels in sharing her world with others. St. John, of course, who takes no notice of Jane's physical appearance, significantly takes no interest at all in this domestic activity. "The humanities and amenities of life had no attraction for him — its peaceful enjoyments no charm" (p. 418).

"It is all very well for the present," he says, "but seriously, I trust when the first flush of vivacity is over, you will look a little higher than domestic endearments and household joys." To which Jane responds simply, that these joys are "the best thing the world has!" There is no direct connection between Jane's establishment in the renovated Moor House and her return to Rochester. But having made her own home there she is free in a way she was not before to return to him and to Thornfield. Moor House, in its "bright, modest snugness," its lack of ostentation and its independence as a self-created world, nicely symbolizes the beauty of her own body that Jane brings to her union with Rochester. As for Thornfield Hall, it had to be burnt down for more reasons than one: Jane never could have converted that imposing pile into a Brontëan nutshell! The smaller manor house of Ferndean, a building "of no architectural pretensions, deep buried in a wood," to which the blind Rochester has retreated after the fire, offers his future wife more scope for a recreation of another private sexual paradise.

The small, scrupulously clean and scrupulously orderly sexual paradise in *Villette* is even more restricted and more exclusively a private world. This is truly a secret place — the tiny "nutshell" of a house, with its adjoining schoolroom, that Monsieur Paul presents to Lucy as his surprise parting gift. And the sexual consummation which is denied at the close of *Villette* is at least symbolically granted in this penultimate vision of Monsieur Paul introducing Lucy to "her" house, which he himself has carefully prepared and equipped exactly to her taste down to its smallest detail. This, then, is a hidden paradise in two senses: hidden from the gaze of the world at large and hidden till now from its own possessor. At the moment of entry Lucy cannot recognize this "pretty place" as her own. The charm of her discovery depends on our knowing not simply the secret she does not yet know (that Monsieur Paul has bought and privately furnished the house and its schoolroom to give to her) but the deeper secret: that as he has made it out of his love for her, he has made it in her own image. And so it is her self, her body, she takes possession of as she enters it with him — in this wonderfully Brontëan version of the discovery scene. It is, again, the world of the "plain and small" revealed as beautiful.

He did not knock, but taking from his pocket a key, he opened and entered at once. Ushering me in, he shut the door behind us. No servant appeared. The vestibule was small, like the house, but freshly and tastefully painted; its vista closed in a French window with vines trailed about the panes, tendrils, and green leaves kissing the glass. Silence reigned in this dwelling . . .

Opening an inner door, M. Paul disclosed a parlour, or salon — very tiny, but I thought, very pretty. Its delicate walls were tinged like a blush; its floor was waxed; a square of brilliant carpet covered its centre; its small round table shone like the mirror over its hearth; there was a little couch, a little chiffoniere; the half-open, crimson-silk door of which, showed porcelain on the shelves; there was a French clock, a lamp; there were ornaments in biscuit china; the re-cess of the single ample window was filled with a green stand, bear-ing three green flower-pots, each filled with a fine plant glowing in bloom; in one corner appeared a gueridon with a marble top, and upon it a work-box, and a glass filled with violets in water. The lat-tice of this room was open; the outer air breathing through, gave freshness, the sweet violets lent fragrance.

"Pretty, pretty place!" said I. M. Paul smiled to see me so pleased.

"Must we sit down here and wait?" I asked in a whisper, half-awed by the deep-pervading hush.

"We will first peep into one or two other nooks of this nut-shell," he replied.

"Dare you take the freedom of going all over the house?" I inquired.

"Yes, I dare," said he, quietly. *(chap. 41, pp. 584–85)*

Whereupon Monsieur Paul takes Lucy into the adjoining school-room and puts a document in her hand which reads, "Externat de demoiselles. Numéro 7, Faubourg Clotilde. Directrice, Mademoi-

selle Lucy Snowe." Monsieur Paul is giving Lucy her professional
independence. But in this scene, which is a proposal scene, he is also
giving her her body — significantly, the two actions are joined. In
part just because they are so joined, Lucy too can see and enjoy the
sexual desirability of her own body — sharing, as it were, in his
curiosity — for this is a new discovery for her as well. As an image
for Lucy's body, this little nutshell of a house takes on a special
weight in *Villette* because it is the only positive image of her person
that we get. Lucy is not Monsieur Paul's "delicate elf" or "mustard-
seed," not, like Jane, "a beauty after [her lover's] own heart, delicate
and aërial." Physical beauty becomes, particularly with this last
heroine, not more qualified, but more hidden, more exclusive of
the world. But what Monsieur Paul sees is for his eyes alone. And
thus it can only be realized for us in the symbolic and private world
of the house to which he alone has the key.

   We should not, I think, forget these tiny, immaculate chambers
in which so much of Brontë's spirit dwells, and dwells in peace —
rooms which inevitably recall the small and plain, the intimately
known and infinitely cared for rooms of Brontë's own home at Haworth parsonage. Theirs is an orderliness that does not mimic the
repressive order of the larger world, but provides a secure setting
for the exercise of feeling — including sexual feeling.

   With the publication in 1979 of Sandra M. Gilbert and Susan
Gubar's now classic work, *The Madwoman in the Attic*, the attic in-
habited by Rochester's mad wife Bertha has become an emblem for
the Victorian woman's frantic effort to escape the airless mansions
of the patriarchal society,[41] as if her only refuge were to retreat,
like Bertha, from the social world to the madness and isolation of
that barren attic chamber. I am suggesting that Brontë, and other
woman writers of her age, have provided us with more than that
— with the image of a place in which a woman may, however precariously or temporarily, discover herself as a sexual person who
can remain true to herself (in *Villette*, for instance, she can have her
adjoining schoolroom) at the same time. Those who would see

Bertha as the suppressed part of Jane's own ego, maddened by a patriarchal world she cannot fight, might note that, in at least one respect — her size — the mad woman of Rochester's attic chamber has more in common with the physical appearance of the hated rival, the society beauty, than she does with Jane herself. When Rochester leads the assembled company up to the attic, what they see there is "a big woman, in stature almost equalling her husband, and corpulent besides" (chap. 26, p. 321). Pointing to the difference between his lunatic wife and "this young girl, who stands so grave and quiet at the mouth of hell," Rochester invites the spectators to compare "this form with that bulk" (p. 322). The madwoman is another incarnation of the imposing, demanding, insatiable woman, all that the self-contained, small and plain, desirable woman repudiates.

To say that Brontë gives us in her fiction those other happier chambers, so nicely suited to her heroines, is not to say that either she or her heroines are secure in their knowledge of themselves as sexually desirable women. The image of the room is just that, an image. What it embodies is a possibility, how this particular woman sees herself as a beautiful, desirable woman — when she can do so. It is an achievement easier to come by in art than in life, but not easy in either sphere. In *Shirley* there is a wonderful, mocking inversion of this whole Brontëan motif of the neat little house as the residence of the neat little sexually desirable woman. The houses of the two virtuous old maids, which the unhappy Caroline visits in her effort to compensate for lost love by throwing herself into a life of good works, are as small and as plain and as "exquisitely clean and neat"[42] as their tenants — and also as barren as the old maids in their "grimly-tidy" persons.[43] The image of those "grimly-tidy" spinsters in their grimly-tidy homes does not give the lie to the images of the Brontëan sexual paradise as we see it in the other novels and elsewhere in *Shirley* as well. It suggests, what Brontë herself must also often have felt in her days of painful solitude at Haworth: how easily is the private paradise converted into the solitary cell! How

precariously thin is the line between the happy welcoming bustle in
the neat little room of one's own and the compulsive tidying-up of
lonely spinsterhood.

In Brontë's own life, there was to be neither the satisfaction of
the sexual paradise into which the adored man is joyfully received
nor, in the end, a lonely spinsterhood. There was instead the marriage to her father's curate, the Reverend Arthur Nicholls. Nicholls
was no intellectual companion for Brontë—no Rochester or
M. Paul Emanuel. It would seem that Brontë agreed to the marriage with Nicholls, where she had refused a number of earlier offers, not out of any sense of desperation for wedlock, but because
she was profoundly moved by the spectacle of a man who could
love her so passionately, so persistently (over a period of some
seven years), and against such large obstacles (her father's jealous
disdain being chief of them). To her old friend Ellen Nussey she
wrote, before the marriage, that "what I taste of happiness is of the
soberest order."[44] Not surprisingly, given such an emotional state,
contemplating her marriage did not make Charlotte Brontë feel
beautiful. To her father, who thought, as Gaskell reports, "she had
a chance of somebody higher or at least farther removed from pov-
erty," she said "Father I am not a young girl, nor a young woman
even (she was thirty-seven)—I never was pretty. I now am ugly.
At your death I will have £300 besides the little I have earned
myself—do you think there are many men who would serve seven
years for me?"[45] Brontë died in March of 1855, it seems due to "normal" complications of a pregnancy which her always frail constitution was not strong enough to bear. According to Nicholls, her
last words to him on her deathbed were, "I am not going to die, am
I? He will not separate us, we have been so happy."[46]

However, the little we know of the final months of Brontë's life
incline me to think that this marriage was not one that could de-
velop (or would have developed, had it continued) the sense of herself as beautiful *as we see it in the novels*. I say this not because the
evidence suggests her marriage was an unhappy one (it doesn't),
but because the marriage was not one that encouraged her full being

to grow and flourish, as must happen in her fiction before beauty is nurtured. In the brief period of her married life the whole tenor of Brontë's letters to her old friends changes dramatically. Excusing her failure to maintain her correspondence with her former school-teacher, she explains, "The fact is my time is not my own now; somebody else wants a good portion of it — and says we must do so and so. We *do* 'so and so' accordingly, and it generally seems the right thing — only I sometimes wish I could have written the letter as well as taken the walk."[47] Written the letter, and perhaps the book . . . ? She confesses in the same letter that she has much less time for thinking now and is obliged to be more practical, for "my dear Arthur is a very practical as well as a very punctual, methodical man." And "now that I am married, I do not expect to be an object of much general interest. Ladies who have won some prominence (call it either *notoriety* or celebrity) in their single life — often fall quite into the back ground when they change their names; but if true domestic happiness replace Fame — the exchange will indeed be for the better." Of course Brontë was wont throughout her life to deprecate whatever gave her pleasure, and particularly her literary ambitions. But now she had someone very close to her to support that tendency toward self-suppression. Brontë's most recent biographer finds it hard to believe that she would not, had she lived, have taken up her writing career after some interval.[48] I find it hard to believe that she would have. Mrs. Gaskell's assertion that "Mr Nicholls always *groaned literally*" when his wife spoke of continuing her fragment of a new novel, *Emma*, written according to her, "a year or so" before Miss Brontë's marriage, may be apocryphal.[49] And the same caveat must be made when quoting Ellen Nussey's recollection of Mr. Nicholls saying he "did not marry Currer Bell, the novelist, but Charlotte Brontë, the clergyman's daughter. Currer Bell may fly to heaven tomorrow for all I care."[50] (Neither woman had reason to feel close sympathy for Nicholls, though Gaskell was the only one of Brontë's friends to give her blessing to the marriage.) Nicholls himself denied in later years that he had ever stood in the way of his wife's literary ambitions.[51] But he certainly did nothing to encourage them. Even if Nussey's recollection of Nicholls's exact words in that last statement is faulty, the dichotomy it assumes between two fictive entities, on the one hand "Currer Bell" — the woman writer in her masculine, public disguise, and on the other hand, "the clergyman's daughter" — the woman as her father's child and perpetuator of his values, stops me in my tracks, since neither pole of that antithesis describes Charlotte Brontë herself — a particular woman and a particular, female novelist.

A few years ago an 1854 photograph was discovered which scholars have good reason to believe is the only extant (and probably the only ever created) photographic image of Charlotte Brontë.[52] I remember my skepticism and dismay when I first saw that image, presumably taken on the Nicholls' honeymoon in Ireland and the companion-piece to a surviving one of her husband. The photograph, shot slightly from below, shows a rounded face and stolid if not unattractive features — its subject, one might conjecture from this image of her upper body, a rather "extensive armful." Brontë, if indeed it is she, is photographed in just slightly more than profile view, gazing perhaps toward the unseen husband, her eyelid modestly lowered. She does not gaze out at the world in this image; the penetrating eyes, so often commented on, and which are the focus of even the softened-up Richmond drawing, do not engage the observer here. "Is it possible," I asked myself, "that this rather plump, bland-looking woman is the real Charlotte Brontë?" I have seen another woman in my mind's eye all these years, an image put together from various surviving sketches, verbal portraits such as I've quoted here, and of course, the testimony of the novels. If this is Charlotte, there's one more proof of the enormity of the gap between "reality" and imagination — everyone's imagination. But on reflection, it seems to me that if this photograph is no Charlotte Brontë *I* can recognize — no defiantly plain woman, no "elf," no "mustard seed," no "beauty just after the desire of my own heart," it might well be a photograph of Mrs. Ar-

thur Nicholls, the curate's wife, a conventionally attractive woman
in the early Victorian mode.

And probably it would be too much to expect that, in her life,
Brontë could have left us with an image of herself such as the one
Gaskell gives us in her biography — an image of one who, both as
a woman and a writer, is fiery and fastidious, passionate and plain.
Enough that Brontë was able to give us those imaginative projections of herself in Jane Eyre and Lucy Snowe, each uniquely pleasing to the singular man who will make the effort to discover the
beauty hidden in the "small and plain" woman and love her for herself. Given all the privations of Brontë's childhood, given the (un-
surprising) unavailability in her own marriageable years of a Rochester or a Paul Emanuel, and given too the strength of her own
impulse for self-sacrifice, it is not surprising if what we are left with
at the end of her life is not the threatened invisibility of the angry
orphan child but the real invisibility of the Victorian matron. We
have, however, the novels.

George Eliot: The Beauty of Presence

*G*eorge Eliot has been a problematic writer for contemporary feminists. Generally agreed to be the greatest English novelist of the late nineteenth century, she is a writer with far greater psychological range than Brontë. In examining the personal, societal, and philosophical issues of her age, she treats (like Shakespeare) the issues of human life in all ages — nothing less than our shared condition. A woman of formidable intellectual powers, who easily held her own among the greatest male thinkers of her day, she was also radical in the choices she made in her own life, redefining the marriage contract in her own terms. She chose not to enter into a clandestine sexual relationship with the man she loved, who was not legally free to divorce the wife who had forsaken him. Had she done so, a society that allowed individuals to do more or less what they wished so long as they kept quiet about it and no one complained, would not have ostracized her. Instead she declared herself Mrs. George Lewes and lived with Lewes openly, while he continued to support his wife and to care for their three sons — as she did also. Thus she forfeited the company of those members of society who could not condone her action (almost all the women and many of the men in her world) and — what cost her a great deal more pain — forfeited any contact with several beloved members of her own family. Eliot's two closest women friends were ardent champions of the movement to put women's education on a par with that of men and extend to them the franchise; and she herself held enlightened views on "the women's issue." How could such a figure, then, not be championed by today's generation of feminists?

Feminists today are indeed drawn to George Eliot; and that is just why many of us feel so frustrated by what she does *not* give us.[1] For the problem is a real one, and the beauty question is close to the center of the difficulty. Eliot is faulted, on the one hand, for giving her heroines too much, for never creating, as Brontë did, a heroine like herself, unblessed with the gift of beauty. And she is faulted, on the other hand, for not giving her heroines enough — for not giving them some equivalent to the emancipated life which she herself enjoyed, both as a writer and a woman whose domestic arrangements defied society. The two criticisms are the two sides of the same coin: instead of giving her heroines lives of action in the larger world, and some hope for reforming that world, she gives them a "consolation prize" — what a narrow, provincial society defines as a better treasure and the thing she herself didn't have: the beauty that wins the admiration of men. The situation is made more poignant because Eliot's most sympathetic heroines, in spirit, *are* like herself: they yearn for meaningful lives beyond the confines of the domestic sphere. Why, then, doesn't she allow them to achieve such lives — and why does she give them the thing she herself deems less worthy? Is the answer to both questions, to put it bluntly, a failure of nerve?

I think that Eliot does, like Brontë, confer on her heroines a beauty that is not unearned but an extension of the personal beauty she came, on some level, to know in herself. I think, then, that her most celebrated heroine — Dorothea Brooke — is, both in her achievements and in the limitations imposed upon her, more like her creator than unlike her. Defined in such terms, this heroine may not, finally, be a congenial figure to some contemporary feminists: whether we admire as well as sympathize with Dorothea in the end depends, for each of us, on how we define a meaningful life. In this chapter I will be describing Eliot's prototypical heroine as I see her (with love), and I will be suggesting why in my own life she has been a valuable model — indeed the most important model of any of the fictional creations discussed in this book.

The argument must focus on Dorothea, the heroine of Eliot's

most ambitious and, most of us would agree, greatest novel, *Mid-dlemarch*, published serially in 1871 and 1872. For it is Dorothea's ardent nature and noble aspirations which are most closely identi-fied with Eliot's own. It is Dorothea to whom readers, over the years, have felt most closely drawn. And it is Dorothea, therefore, who provokes the greatest frustration. Her beauty, we may notice, is the subject of the novel's very first sentence: "Miss Brooke had that kind of beauty which seems to be thrown into relief by poor dress."[2] I want, however, to begin not at that starting point but with a scene that takes place about one-quarter of the way into the novel. As *Middlemarch* is an unusually long novel even by nineteenth-century standards, that takes us fairly far into the action. A bit of background, then: Dorothea, a wealthy and high-minded but typ-ically undereducated young woman of the early nineteenth cen-tury, longs to do something with her life that will enrich the exis-tence of others and therefore her own. But what might that something be? She meets an austere scholar, Edward Casaubon, some twenty years older than she, and imagines that a marriage with him will answer her hopes. A man wholly dedicated to a great life-work, he is different from the idle, affable gentry folk among whom she has been reared: she will help him in whatever way she can to further the work whose publication much enriches us all. Shortly before her marriage she briefly meets the disinherited young relation whose education her future husband is funding, Will Ladislaw — a young man of about her own age, interested in the arts but uncertain as to what vocation he might pursue. And it is through Will's eyes that we first see Dorothea after her marriage, on her honeymoon in Rome: Casaubon is pursuing his scholarly research; she is making the usual tour of the great monuments to the city's heritage. The scene is the Vatican gallery; Will and his artist-friend, Naumann, are viewing the treasures of the great gal-lery together, when the latter man's eye is caught by the spectacle not of an object of art, but of another spectator. It is Dorothea (with whom Naumann has no way of knowing his friend is acquainted), and Naumann calls out to Will, "Come here, quick! else she will have changed her pose!" (chap. 19, p. 219).

In the portrait which then follows, Dorothea is seen through the eyes of the two friends, and by the reader who has not seen her in some time — but seen as an object of the artists' gaze (Will himself was introduced to us in the earlier scene in England with a sketch book in his hand). And she is seen as she stands looking at an art-object herself, to which we are invited by the masculine spectator to compare her: it is a statue of "the reclining Ariadne, then called the Cleopatra." The configuration vividly recalls the Cleopatra scene in *Villette*, where Lucy looks disparagingly at the painting of the half-naked Cleopatra. In both scenes a Protestant heroine, clothed in "Quakerish grey," looks at a pagan art object displayed in an alien Catholic country: a figure of a naked woman whose blatant sexuality creates (as Naumann puts it) "a fine bit of antithesis" with her own figure — an antithesis which is in turn appreciated by a man who gazes at *her*. For in the *Villette* scene M. Emanuel has spied Lucy gazing at the Cleopatra painting and quickly draws her away from a subject he sees as unfit for a young woman's eyes. In the Brontë scene, as in Eliot's, the essential message to be gained from the spectacle of the female observer of the Cleopatra who is herself observed by her future lover is that he would rather look at *her*. The parallels are close enough to make me think that Eliot is consciously invoking here a scene from a novel whose merits she was quick to appreciate.[3] The similarities present us with a nice opportunity to contrast Eliot's treatment with Brontë's — of a particular motif and of the beauty question generally as it is handled by the two women novelists. Here, then, is Eliot's portrait:

> Quickness was ready at the call, and the two figures passed lightly
> along by the Meleagers toward the hall where the reclining Ar-
> iadne, then called the Cleopatra, lies in the marble voluptuousness
> of her beauty, the drapery folding around her with a petal-like ease
> and tenderness. They were just in time to see another figure stand-
> ing against a pedestal near the reclining marble: a breathing bloom-

ing girl, whose form, not shamed by the Ariadne, was clad in
Quakerish grey drapery; her long cloak, fastened at the neck, was
thrown backward from her arms, and one beautiful ungloved hand
pillowed her cheek, pushing somewhat backward the white beaver
bonnet which made a sort of halo to her face around the simply
braided dark-brown hair. She was not looking at the sculpture,
probably not thinking of it: her large eyes were fixed dreamily
on a streak of sunlight which fell across the floor. *(chap. 19,
pp. 219–20)*

Do you feel some uneasiness reading this passage? Does it seem as
though Eliot is pulling us right back into the old patriarchal way of
gazing at the woman's body? Insisting that she hold her pose?
Seeing her as an art object rather than as a real person? Whatever
your response, you will agree, I think, comparing Eliot's portrait
to its counterpart in *Villette*, that Eliot greatly narrows the gap between the "breathing blooming,", erect, Protestant young woman
and her painted (or in this case sculpted) "antithesis." In the first
place, Dorothea, as well as the Cleopatra, is "composed" for us in
this tableau: by Will who, unwittingly, is beginning to fall in love
with Dorothea; by his artist-friend Naumann; and by the author
herself, who looks at her subject both as an artist and as a lover. It
is Dorothea, not the pagan goddess, who is now the first object of
both sexual and aesthetic scrutiny. She is the one whom the observers have crossed the corridor to see. It is she who, "not shamed by
the Ariadne," receives the extended portrait; the Ariadne herself
gets only a line. And Dorothea can, so to speak, stand the comparison. Her Quakerish grey dress is metamorphosed into "Quakerish
grey *drapery*"; and in an unreligious age, her beaver bonnet is trans-
formed into the halo of devotion — Will's devotion.

Furthermore, if Dorothea herself is more like an art-object here,
the figured Cleopatra is also more like the "breathing blooming
woman." For we are invited here, as we emphatically were not in
Villette, to enjoy the Cleopatra's sexuality, which is infused with a
tenderness which might almost be said to have been borrowed from
Dorothea herself. Voluptuous sensuality and a "petal-like ease and

tenderness" coexist here in harmony, as they never do in Brontë's world. For it is not only the Cleopatra's sexual nature we enjoy; it is also Dorothea's. In fact, in a striking reversal of the Brontëan antithesis, here it is the antique beauty whose drapery-attire is folded protectively about her, while Dorothea is seen in the gesture of freeing herself from the confinement of dress: the Quakerish cloak is thrown backward to expose her arms; the hat too is pushed somewhat backward; and she has removed the glove from her hand. Not that there is any hint of a sexual invitation in Dorothea's "pose," but her whole stance implies the presence of a sexuality which is, like the Cleopatra's, an acknowledged part of her beauty. Or, to put it somewhat differently, the bedroom associations of that "one beautiful ungloved hand *pillowed* on her cheek" do not seem at odds with the pensiveness which informs her whole posture, as she stands, lost in her own thoughts. In more ways than one, then, this portrait might be said to command from us the response solicited on behalf of another unabashedly sexual Cleopatra by Shakespeare's Enobarbus: "Kneel down, kneel down, and wonder."

But what, finally, are we being asked to admire here? Shouldn't Dorothea *do* something to command such devotion, not just stand there looking at once saintlike and desirable? It is the old uneasiness: beauty seeming to demand a devotion it has not *earned*. And we may feel it all the more acutely here, just because Dorothea's beauty is so laden with the promise of virtuous action. But a promise is not the same as the thing itself; gestures are not actions. And the "movement and tone" that in his subsequent exchange with Naumann Will insists are more divine than the "mere coloured superficies" (which is all Naumann can see when he looks admiringly at Dorothea with his painterly eyes), are still not to be confused with deeds and words. Is there on Eliot's own part an effort to persuade us to take the first as a substitute for the second? Does Eliot perhaps make so much of Dorothea's "beautiful ungloved hand" as a way of deflecting our attention away from the fact that, as a helping hand, it does not accomplish so much in the end? The model houses for the workers Dorothea dreams of never do get built. And closer to home, those whom she would most wish to save — Casaubon, Rosamond, above all, Lydgate, the most redeemable — are not saved. If Dorothea had done more, would Eliot have "needed" to pay so much attention to the beauty of her hand? Surely there is some relation between all those apparitions in the novel of Dorothea's beautiful person and Eliot's retrospective portrait in the novel's "Finale" of a life whose "determining acts . . . were *not* ideally beautiful" (p. 896).

There is a relation, and one I want to say more about. But first let us look back once more at the portrait, for there are important ways in which it departs from, even radically resists, being placed within the category of all those imprisoning masculine gazes which rightly make us uneasy. For one thing, to the extent that the masculine viewers may be placing themselves in that tradition, Dorothea herself resists playing the woman's conventional role in the familiar drama. In asking his friend to come quickly, "before she changes her pose," Naumann acknowledges that the "breathing blooming" woman has a freedom the statue does not possess. And in fact Dorothea exercises that freedom in the line immediately following the ones I have just quoted: "But she became conscious of the two strangers who suddenly paused as if to contemplate the Cleopatra, and, without looking at them, immediately turned away to join a maid-servant and courier who were loitering along the hall at a little distance off." Second, though in the portrait itself I think we are seeing Dorothea essentially through Will's eyes, those of the lover-to-be, in the subsequent interchange between the two men Will refuses to play the accustomed role of co-conspirator. When Naumann goes on, spinning out an increasingly intellectualized rhapsody on "the most perfect young Madonna I ever saw," and (when Will tells him of his relation to her) suggests Will persuade his wealthy cousin to have his wife's portrait taken by himself, Will finds himself becoming indignant and oddly defensive on Dorothea's behalf, though he hardly knows her. To Naumann's statement that if Will himself were a true artist he would agree with everything he has just said on the subject of Dorothea's beauty, Will responds, "Yes, and that your painting her was the chief outcome of her existence" (chap. 19, p. 221), thus exposing the egotism that underlies centuries of patriarchal gazing. And, Will continues, becoming increasingly heated,

> And what is a portrait of a woman? Your painting and Plaskic are poor stuff after all. They perturb and dull conceptions instead of raising them. Language is a finer medium . . .
>
> Language gives a fuller image, which is all the better for being vague. After all, the true seeing is within; and painting stares at you with an insistent imperfection. I feel that especially about representations of women. As if a woman were a mere coloured superficies! You must wait for movement and tone. There is a difference in their very breathing: they change from moment to moment. — This woman whom you have just seen, for example: how would you paint her voice, pray? But her voice is much diviner than anything you have seen of her.   *(chap. 19, p. 222)*

Of course Ladislaw (and Eliot) are following the prescription Eliot expressed in the very action of defending it: offering us the "fuller image" that language (the writer's medium) can bring — in part through its refusal to pin down the image, to reduce the woman to "a coloured superficies." In words which stress the importance of movement and change, as well as of voice, Ladislaw (and Eliot) fill out, or revise, Naumann's portrait in the mode of the women writers who bring to their heroine-portraiture this same awareness that "the true seeing is within." At the end of this scene, Will, leaving the gallery, wonders why he has been getting so irritated, why he should make "any fuss about Mrs Casaubon? And yet he felt as if something had happened to him with regard to her" (pp. 222–23).

What has happened? Will had seen Dorothea before, prior to her marriage, and had not been particularly impressed by her — though he had been taken with her voice.[4] I think Will discovers Dorothea's beauty here, and begins to discover his love for her, because what he perceives intuitively when he looks at her is the frustration with her marriage and the desire to escape from its prison-house she doesn't yet know she feels. As we will learn in the next chapter, all Dorothea feels is a vague confusion and discontent which focuses on a disappointment with the eternal city. She doesn't yet suspect that the object of her disenchantment is Mr. Casaubon, that it is her marriage, not the holy city, in which she is beginning to lose faith. And of course Will doesn't know this either — though he will know it two hours later when he goes to call on Dorothea and sees the evidence of recent tears on her face: he will understand better than she can yet the source of those tears. And, just because the true seeing *is* within, he can see all this, or intuit it, not only before she does, but before we do. For it is all there in the portrait scene (though Naumann sees none of it). It is there in the pensiveness of her posture and the abstraction of her gaze, directed at that streak of sunlight on the floor — as if to follow its source out into the open air of freedom. And it is there in the way her outer clothing is pushed aside, as if in an impulse to free herself from constriction. Will sees Dorothea as beautiful now, as not before, because now he can read feelings in her to which his heart goes out.

The two indexes for beauty in Eliot's fiction, and in her own person, are the two things Will singles out here in his reproach to Naumann: movement and voice. Ultimately, the two overlap, as both are aspects of expressiveness, but let me discuss them separately. First, movement.

Where the small Brontë heroine "shrinks" in her corner, fearing invisibility but hoping to be seen and loved, the large Eliot heroine never assumes a posture of hiding. She is always, like her creator, a large, conspicuous figure. Marian Evans, before her union with George Lewes, saw herself as conspicuously ugly. In a series of letters written to her friends the Brays when she was in her early thirties, and when an intense relationship with the philosopher Herbert Spencer was much on her mind and much in question, she called herself "a hideous hag,"[5] "haggard as an old witch,"[6] "like one of those old hags we used to see by the wayside in Italy — only a little worse, for want of the dark eyes and dark hair in contrast with the parchment."[7] Four years later, in 1856, she saw some other "hideous hags," two cockle women glimpsed on another foreign wayside. But her traveling companion was George Lewes now, and she had recently made the most momentous decision of her life, to live openly with him. The "hideous hags" have become powerfully expressive figures. One of the two women, she says in her *Recollections* of this momentous journey, "was the grandest woman I ever saw — six feet high, carrying herself like a Greek Warrior, and treading the earth with unconscious majesty. They wore large woolen shawls of a rich brown, doubled lengthwise, with the end thrown back again over the left shoulder so as to fall behind in graceful folds."[8]

Dorothea does not, as we saw her in the Vatican gallery, assume the posture of a Greek Warrior. But the image of the garment unconsciously removed or thrown back, of the human form (the "breathing blooming girl") boldly declaring itself — as if to break through the constrictions not just of dress but of the whole social edifice of form which dress may symbolize — becomes the signature of Eliot's heroine of difficult beauty. The recurrent notice Eliot pays throughout her fiction to women who somehow manage to look beautiful in spite of the (always) abominable and (generally) constricting fashions of an earlier era — from Milly Barton and Janet Dempster, in her first published fiction, the three stories compromising the *Scenes of Clerical Life*,[9] to Nancy Lammeter in *Silas Marner*,[10] all the way through to the end — is not just a "window dressing" cue to period style. These descriptions are given so that we may see the Eliot heroine's beauty as the emergence of the powerful inner self through gestures of self-expression and communication. Even the beautiful dairy maid, Hetty Sorrel, in Eliot's first novel, *Adam Bede* (1859), a bad girl who doesn't "deserve" this sort of treatment, gets it anyway: "her curly hair, though all pushed back under her round cap while she was at work, stole back in dark delicate rings on her forehead and about her white shell-like ears," and "the linen butter-making apron, with its bib, seemed a thing to be imitated in silk by duchesses, since it fell in such charming lines,

[and] her brown stockings and thick-soled shoes lost all that clumsiness which they must certainly have had when empty of her foot and ankle."[11] This has its not so distant kinship to the beauty of Dorothea Brooke which "was thrown into relief" by poor dress — even though the "poor dress" Dorothea might wear would be a wealthy woman's garment of choice while Hetty's is forced upon her.

We see Maggie Tulliver in *The Mill on the Floss* (1860) "throw[ing] her bonnet off very carelessly and coming in with her hair rough as well as out of curl."[12] In the remainder of the paragraph, Eliot develops the contrast we have come to expect between the heroine's latent beauty and the more obvious beauty of a prettier (but not really prettier) rival, Maggie and her cousin Lucy. Eliot makes it a contrast between motion and stasis as well as between the large woman and the small one. Where Maggie comes rushing in, Lucy stands quietly, "in her natty completeness," by her mother's knee — and waits patiently, as it were, for her features to be catalogued — from her "neatest little rosebud mouth" which she holds up to be kissed, to her "little round neck with the row of coral beads," her "little straight nose," and her "little clear eyebrows." In Eliot's fiction both the heroine and her rival are the physical opposites to their counterparts in Brontë: in Eliot it is the heroine who undoes her constricting clothing as she moves toward her interlocutor; her rival who remains quiet, covered up. Each has a different task to perform — Eliot's heroine reaches out toward us in an act of sympathetic communication; Brontë's remains aloof until she is met on her own terms, discovered and loved.

Everywhere in Eliot's fiction we see the heroine's outstretched hand and arm. Dorothea never "gives" her hand to a man as we would expect a woman of her station in this age to do — a vestige of the old custom in which a woman gives her hand in order to receive the homage of a kiss. Dorothea "holds out" her hand to Ladislaw in Rome, "puts out" her hand to Lydgate at Lowick — a small difference in terminology but expressive of the difference between the passive gesture and the active one, in which the heart's offerings go out with the hand. Celia, Dorothea's younger sister and one of two "other women" in this novel (and though very different from one another, both drawn in the terms of the patriarchal convention) uses her hands as containers, taking "habitual care of whatever she held in her hands" (chap. 5, p. 72), while Dorothea's — like her creator's — "not thin hands, or small hands; but powerful, feminine, maternal hands" (chap. 4, p. 61) reach out to divest themselves of ownership.

A scene in *The Mill on the Floss*, in which the heroine's extended arm plays a crucial role in the action of the plot, may help us better understand the charge that beauty carries in Eliot's fictional world and its possible complications. We have already seen the groundwork laid for the large, unruly Maggie's rivalry with and eventual triumph over her cousin Lucy in that opening scene. Some time before that victory (with its disastrous consequences) actually occurs, Maggie protests when her friend Philip teasingly predicts Maggie's ultimate victory over her cousin Lucy in a contest for the desirable male: "As if I, with my old gowns, and want of all accomplishments, could be a rival of dear little Lucy, who knows and does all sorts of charming things, and is ten times prettier than I am — even if I were odious and base enough to wish to be her rival" (bk. 5, chap. 4, p. 433). But we know, if Maggie doesn't quite, just how much mere "prettiness," even prettiness multiplied ten times over, counts in Eliot's world: about as much as the new clothes and the superficial feminine accomplishments in which "little Lucy" has been schooled! Then, just prior to the fatal denouement, Lucy herself says to Maggie, "*I* can't think what witchery it is in you, Maggie, that makes you look best in shabby clothes. . . . Now if I were to put anything shabby on, I should be quite unnoticeable — I should be a mere rag" (bk. 6, chap. 2, p. 480).

Yes. The shabby clothes do display the Eliot heroine at her best, for they provide the maximum field of resistance for her gestures toward self-assertion. Yet Maggie's anxiety is real, not merely coy. She senses that her beauty, as an extension of her own self and her long pent-up desires, has the power to bring pain as well as pleasure. And she is right. As no more an "ugly duckling" but a beautiful swan now, carried away by a yearning for a love she has never received at home, Maggie allows herself to be seduced by Stephen Guest — understood to be all-but-engaged to Lucy, but infatuated with Maggie. Both Maggie and Stephen are present at a large dance and, without exactly willing it to happen, have drawn apart from the others and drifted into the conservatory, where Maggie looks at the flowers and Stephen looks at her.

> Stephen was mute: he was incapable of putting a sentence together, and Maggie bent her arm a little upward toward the large half-opened rose that had attracted her. Who has not felt the beauty of a woman's arm? — the unspeakable suggestions of tenderness that lie in the dimpled elbow and all the varied gently lessening curves down to the delicate wrist with its tiniest, almost imperceptible nicks in the firm softness.   (bk. 6, chap. 10, p. 561)

The gesture is a very maternal one, and its appeal for Eliot may be rooted in the way it combines the impulse of tenderness with that of mastery. In Maggie the two impulses are not yet wholly fused. Her beauty, like that of all Eliot heroines, is realized in a movement of self-extension; but the action is not without predatory overtones. Maggie has just said to Stephen, "I think I am quite wicked with roses — I like to gather them and smell them till they have no scent left." If the scene symbolizes the act of sexual deflowering, we must be struck by the fact that it is Maggie and not Stephen who is plucking the rose. The large Eliot heroine tends, however covertly, to usurp the sexual initiative from the man. Yet as Stephen continues gazing mutely at Maggie's arm, an authorial digression superimposes upon the rose-plucking image a second one, in which the outstretched arm reaches not to pluck a flower but, in a gesture of love, toward a fellow human being: "A woman's arm touched the soul of a great sculptor two thousand years ago, so that he wrought an image of it for the Parthenon which moves us still as it clasps lovingly the time-worn marble of a headless trunk. Maggie's was such an arm as that — and it had the warm tints of life" (p. 561).

Here is Eliot's resolution — in the image of a love that can outlast the disintegration of its object, or of a love which, like Maggie's for Stephen, is finer than its object merits. Maggie is on her way to becoming the mature Eliot heroine, whose beauty is defined in the powerful maternal act of love given to one weaker than herself.[13] But Maggie has not fully achieved that stage, and she never will do so. Frightened by that part of herself — the insufficiently loved part of herself — which would still rather extend her power *over* the man than extend it *to* him, in a familiar dynamic of Western sexual politics Maggie ends up by surrendering her power and her identity altogether.

Marian Evans (George Eliot) never "stole" a man away from a helpless rival. But many members of her society certainly saw her illegal union with Lewes in such terms. And what if that "other woman" had not already abandoned the desired man for another by whom she had already borne at least two children? Might Marian Evans, so long admired as "Clematis," or "*mental* beauty,"[14] so belatedly loved in the flesh, had the circumstances of her own situation been somewhat different, not possibly have acted as Maggie acts? And having done so, might she too not have made such a "suicidal" retreat as Maggie then makes, back to the first family which had rejected her and valued neither her mental nor her physical beauty? Beauty, in Eliot's world, is associated with sexual power in a way it is not in Brontë's. And sexual power, as we all know, has its dangerous side — especially for one who has long felt powerless. In *The Mill on the Floss* Eliot plays out a situation that might have been her own fate.

By the time she wrote *Middlemarch*, ten years after *The Mill on the Floss*, Eliot's own yearning for the power beauty confers on a woman over a man had been assuaged. Her relationship with Lewes had all the marks of long-established and self-renewing domesticity; she was also a beloved "Mutter" to his three sons. In the dramatic climaxes of *Middlemarch*, where the heroine's beauty is again epitomized by her outstretched arm and hand, such actions have been purged of any predatory overtones; and what is left is the maternal gesture, the expression of a desire to extend oneself to another whose need is greater than one's own. Not long after the scene in the Vatican gallery, when Casaubon and Dorothea have returned to England and he has (sadly) learned to fear the ardor of the wife they both thought would be his devoted and unquestioning helpmate, that hand goes out poignantly to the husband who cannot reciprocate the gesture: "Mr Casaubon kept his hands behind him and allowed her pliant arm to cling with difficulty against his rigid arm" (chap. 42, p. 462). Near the end of the novel it goes out to Ladislaw, who can reciprocate it: "and so they stood, with their hands clasped, like two children, looking out on the storm. . . . Then they turned their faces towards each other, with the memory of his last words in them, and they did not lose each other's hands" (chap. 83, p. 868). And in the encounter which constitutes the emotional if not the romantic climax of *Middlemarch*, Dorothea extends her large hand to her rival's small one. The beautiful Rosamond, who has herself just made a bid for Ladislaw's affection which Dorothea does not yet know was unreciprocated, at first resists but then accepts Dorothea's offering of love and forgiveness — as the small woman's reflex gesture of self-protection is met by the other's of self-exposure, and the one woman's protective putting on of superfluous clothing by the other's taking off of the same:

> Rosamond, wrapping her soft shawl around her as she walked towards Dorothea, was inwardly wrapping her soul in cold reserve. . . . Looking like the lovely ghost of herself, her graceful slimness wrapped in her soft white shawl, the rounded infantine mouth and cheek inevitably suggesting mildness and innocence, Rosamond paused at three yards' distance from her visitor and bowed. But Dorothea, who had taken off her gloves, from an impulse which she could never resist when she wanted a sense of freedom, came forward, and with her face full of a sad yet sweet openness, put out her hand. Rosamond could not avoid meeting her glance, could not avoid putting her small hand into Dorothea's which clasped it with gentle motherliness. *(chap. 81, pp. 850–51)*

But of course Eliot was not simply Lewes's beloved wife, his sexual and intellectual partner, and an important mother-figure for his sons. She was a great novelist. So we must address the question of what she does *not* give her heroines. This is where Will's emphasis on the beauty of Dorothea's *voice* is relevant. For Eliot, beauty, as it is an extension of oneself in space toward another, is an action of communication, a form of expressiveness or eloquence; beauty is the capacity to "say," if only through a look, all that is in one's heart. Eliot has been accused of being cruelly vindictive to the beautiful but heartless Hetty at the end of *Adam Bede*, the ugly woman "punishing" the beautiful one for having what she herself does not have.[15] But what is remarkable to me is how *much* Eliot gives Hetty — or the value she places on her beauty.

Unlike Brontë, Eliot does not punish her "other women" by belittling their beauty or relegating its effects to a superficial sensuality. Eliot gives Hetty's beauty all that it would have if it were *her own* beauty: and that is, above all, the power to express a capacity for love. (This is why Hetty's heavy clothing has the same expressive power that dull or oppressive clothing confers on Eliot's "true" heroines, even though Hetty's clothing has no "right" to send out such signals.) So Hetty's seducer, Arthur Donnithorne, never feels more drawn to her than when, having decided he must forego his passion for the girl and passing her by on the dance floor, he *imagines* he sees an expression of pain on her face. He is mistaken: the pale look on Hetty's face "was only the sign of the struggle between the desire for him to notice her, and the dread lest she should betray the desire to others" (chap. 26, p. 330). Or, Eliot continues, mistaken and yet not mistaken, for "Hetty's face had a language that transcended her feelings. There are faces which nature charges with a meaning and pathos not belonging to the single human soul that flutters beneath them, but speaking the joys and sorrows of foregone generations — eyes that tell of deep love which doubtless has been and is somewhere, but not paired with those eyes — perhaps paired with pale eyes that can say nothing; just as a national language may be instinct with poetry unfelt by the lips that use it." It is an extraordinary notion. Hetty, incapable of deep feeling for another, becomes the possessor, as it were, of a recessive gene for emotions she herself knows nothing of. Eliot develops this same idea more fully in a later passage where she justifies the good Adam's love for the beautiful, soulless Hetty on this same ground. Is it a weakness, she asks rhetorically, to be moved by exquisite music?

> If not, then neither is it a weakness to be so wrought upon by the exquisite curves of a woman's cheek and neck and arms, by the liquid depths of her beseeching eyes, or the sweet childish pout of her lips. . . . Beauty has an expression beyond and far above the one woman's soul that it clothes . . . it is more than a woman's love that moves us in a woman's eyes — it seems to be a far-off mighty love that has come near to us, and made speech for itself there; the rounded neck, the dimpled arm, move us by something more than their prettiness — by their close kinship with all we have known of tenderness and peace.   *(chap. 33, pp. 399–400)*

It *is* an extraordinary notion, a measure of the homage Eliot pays in this first novel to the beauty that is only skin deep — the homage of refusing to leave it at that. The metaphor of beauty as language runs through these passages: beauty is love that has "made speech for itself"; it is being able to articulate and share all that is in one's heart. Ugliness, then, is not so much the sense of feeling oneself unnoticed or uncared for (as in Brontë) but a failure in communication, a sense that one's face can not "speak" all the love that is in one's heart; ugliness is pale eyes — the pale eyes of Eliot's own young womanhood? — that can say nothing. In an earlier scene in *Adam Bede* Adam sees Hetty feeding some baby chicks and (like Donnithorne) falsely attributes to her all sorts of tender emotions — in this instance maternal ones. The narrator comments: "Molly, the housemaid, with a turn-up nose and a protuberant jaw, was really a tenderhearted girl, and, as Mrs Poyser said, a jewel to look after the poultry, but her stolid face showed nothing of this maternal delight, any more than a brown earthenware pitcher will show the light of the lamp within it" (chap. 15, p. 200).

To be ugly is to feel the impulses of one's heart thus blocked, trapped by a barrier which prevents one's feelings from being known by or shared with others. If the clothing which drapes the body of the beautiful woman yields to the pressure from within, the brown earthenware jug, the ugly woman's exterior, blunts it. For Eliot the greatest threat is of being denied the capacity to make one's feelings known—above all, to be denied speech, persuasive speech, the medium, for her, of both love and art. This is perhaps why, in her fiction, the most potent sexual act is not (as generally in Victorian fiction) the meeting of mouths, which is an action for Eliot too suggestive of speech stopped. Instead, as I have already suggested, it is rather the union of hands. Thus, when Rosamond and Dorothea part, at the close of the interview whose initial gestures on each side we have already seen — and part after a true opening of their hearts to one another—Dorothea once more "put[s] out her hand" to Rosamond, "and they said an earnest, quiet good-bye without kiss or other show of effusion: there had been between them too much serious emotion for them to use the signs of it superficially" (chap. 81, p. 858). In Eliot's fiction the handclasp signifies *more* than the expected kiss would have implied.

In *Adam Bede*, Eliot reanimates and puts to rest the haunting fantasy (or paired fantasies) of her young womanhood. For after *Adam Bede* there are no more Hetty Sorrels in her fiction, and there are no more pale eyes that can say nothing. The conventional beauty of Gwendolyn Harleth, in Eliot's last novel, *Daniel Deronda* (1876), is not seductive in the sense that Hetty's is, promising something it cannot deliver, "speaking" to us of more feeling than it knows. Despite the series of question marks about Gwendolyn's beauty which punctuate the opening paragraphs of that novel,[16] her beauty has no real mystery to it and arouses no real curiosity in us. Which is how it should be. For Gwendolyn's beauty *is* gratuitous, separate from herself. And interestingly, Eliot, now that she herself understands this truth, allows Gwendolyn to realize it too. Looking at herself in the mirror, Gwendolyn sees how her beauty is not something she can have any power over; others must like it, because if they don't, she has no power to change it.[17] And we know, with Gwendolyn, the sadness of such a merely external beauty: "Strange and piteous to think what a centre of wretchedness a delicate piece of human flesh like that might be, wrapped round with fine raiment, her ears pierced for gems, her head held loftily, her mouth all smiling pretence, the poor soul within her sitting in sick distaste of all things" (chap. 35, p. 466). Here Gwendolyn's clothing does not yield to the pressure of her form; the ears pierced for gems suggest a kind of beauty that wounds the body it adorns; Gwendolyn's clothing, like Rosamond's, is imagined as a wrapping, something that might protect or hide the body within it — as, on a deeper level, the flesh hides and ultimately betrays the spirit trapped within it. But Eliot feels less wonder for Gwendolyn, she feels more sympathy than she could for Hetty. She is kinder to Gwendolyn than to Rosamond too — not forcing her to compete with a Dorothea. Ironically, Gwendolyn is ultimately humanized by that pitiful soul cowering within her, and having been so, can become beautiful in Eliot's own mold: "Mrs Grandcourt was handsomer than Gwendolyn Harleth: her grace and expression were informed by a greater variety of inward experience." She has become, as Eliot says, "more fully a human being" (chap. 54, p. 741).

Eliot exorcises the fantasy of the beauty which speaks of more than it knows by paying tribute to it in the portrait of Hetty Sorrel, but also by the act of writing the novel, which is itself the greatest possible proof of its creator's own eloquence. Perhaps once one is assured one *can* find a medium in which to speak persuasively to others of "the joys and sorrows of foregone generations" not with the eyes but with the tongue, then it seems more possible, not to forego the eloquence of eyes but to believe in one's own capacity to speak with that other kind of eloquence as well.

The beauty of Eliot's own speaking voice is the first thing John Cross, the husband of her last year (after Lewes's death), recalls in describing his own meeting with her: "through the dimness of these fifteen years and all that has happened in them, I still seem to hear, as I first heard then, the low, earnest, deep musical tones of her voice."[18] The young Henry James's wonderful portrait of the "magnificently ugly — deliciously hideous" George Eliot concludes with a tribute to the "powerful beauty" which resides "in this vast ugliness," and "which, in a very few minutes steals forth and charms the mind, so that you end as I ended, in falling in love with her. . . . I don't know in what the charm lies, but it is thoroughly potent. An admirable physiognomy — a delightful expression, a voice soft and rich as that of a counselling angel . . .'"[19] So I surmise it was not only Lewes's love that allowed Eliot to know her own beauty, but his love combined with the discovery of her own fictional voice — the one releasing the other. And it would seem that this beauty "came through" to those with whom she felt in sympathy.[20] She became, in time, no longer a woman "whose pale eyes could say nothing."

What though, of what Eliot does *not* give her heroines — the life of action in the world which she herself knew? Dorothea's "full nature," in *Middlemarch*'s concluding simile, "like that river of which Cyrus broke the strength, spent itself in channels which had no great name on the earth" (p. 896). The image of the conqueror who *breaks* the strength of the river, speaks for the power of a social tyranny which offers very limited outlets for even the most substantive, rarest woman's talents. The current of the river is diffused — not blocked — however. Unlike that of her creator, Dorothea's life will not be that of a celebrity; unlike Eliot's, her body will lie in an unmarked and (eventually) an unvisited grave. But what, of real importance, I ask myself, is lost here? Eliot may have enjoyed her notoriety, particularly in the later years; and I am sure she enjoyed the actual exercise of her talents. But just as Dorothea's "finely-touched spirit had still its fine issues, though they were not widely visible," would not the "fine issues" — the *effect* of her work on us — incalculably large as it is diffuse — have mattered most to Eliot? I like to think so.

Perhaps I can best suggest that effect by trying to define what it is this beautiful Eliot heroine gives us — the ideal that has been a valuable model in my life — and what she cannot give us. The difference might best be expressed in terms of a distinction between the power of presence and the power of action. Dorothea has the one kind of power but not the other. Her gestures are not "empty

gestures"; but the emphasis on gesture rather than on deed helps define the nature of her power and its limitations. "What is it you
gentlemen are thinking of when you are with Mrs Casaubon?"
Rosamond asks Will. And he responds, "Herself. . . . When one
sees a perfect woman, one never thinks of her attributes — one is
conscious of her presence" (p. 473). What, we may ask, is the good
of being there, if one can't do anything? (As I have already noted,
the model houses do not get built; Rosamond's opening up of herself
to Dorothea is but a momentary opening — she will close up quickly
enough and remain closed in the end; Lydgate's life is not redeemed
by Dorothea's presence — as much as she would wish it to be.

What good then is presence? My answer is, a lot. Being there for
another person is, in the last analysis, all we can ever *do* for one another anyway. A great novelist, for instance, cannot make changes
happen in our lives. He or she can only give us an offering, a sug-
gestion of how things might be; whether we see it or take it up
must, in the end, be our own responsibility. When Lydgate in his
great need opens his heart to Dorothea, he sees her face looking up
at him and discovers how "the presence of a noble nature, generous
in its wishes, ardent in its charity, changes the light for us" (chap.
76, p. 819). Dorothea does not save Lydgate; she does not even have
any very useful advice to offer him. All she really does is show him
that she believes in the power of his own best self — which is, we
might note, the most important thing that a parent gives to a child.
And so, for that moment, Dorothea's presence changes the light for
Lydgate.

Eliot describes the relation between beauty and presence most
clearly and perhaps most eloquently in her last novel, *Daniel Deronda*, where again we see not simply what the beautiful woman
gives but what she gives back to us: namely our faith in ourselves.
The woman in question is Catherine Arrowpoint, a seemingly
plain "difficult" beauty, who wins the true devotion of a man
which Gwendolyn never does. Her Klesmer is a pianist, a man of
no great means, who falls in love (to everyone's surprise) with his
student Catherine, herself an heiress. Who would have thought she

would notice him, when he lacks the prerequisite masculine attribute: social standing. And who would have thought he would notice her, when she lacks the prerequisite feminine one: beauty. Eliot comments:

> Outsiders might have been more apt to think that Klesmer's position was dangerous for himself if Miss Arrowpoint had been an acknowledged beauty; not taking into account that the most powerful of all beauty is that which reveals itself after sympathy and not before it. There is a charm of eye and lip which comes with every little phrase that certifies delicate perception or fine judgment, with every unostentatious word or smile that shows a heart awake to others; and no sweep of a garment or turn of a figure is more satisfying than that which enters as a restoration of confidence that one person is *present* on whom no intention will be lost.[21]   *(chap. 22, p. 281, my italics)*

Some of us might prefer to see more power in the life, the power of a Saint Theresa, and less in the person, less presence. Readers who do not like all the paeons to Dorothea's beauty in *Middlemarch* which, as I have been suggesting, are tributes to the power of her presence, do not like the ending of the novel either (or do not like it if they read it rightly, as an affirmation rather than an acknowledgement of failure), do not like it that we should be asked to admire a life of imperfect fulfillment in the world. They are two kinds of satisfaction, two kinds of power. As the ending of *Middlemarch* makes unequivocally clear, Eliot understood very well the difference between the two and also valued both, as they should be valued. But of the two kinds, I think it is the power of presence she admired the most, the kind of power she gives to Dorothea, a power closer to the novelist's own power — of an eloquence that cannot change our lives but can only be there for us. It is the kind I admire most too.

CHAPTER 6

Two Mastectomy Narratives:
Beauty and Body-Integrity

*I*f our bodies speak eloquently of who we are and how we feel about ourselves, then what does it mean for a woman to lose that part of her body which is the visible symbol of her identity as a woman — her breast? It means she is not simply faced with a threat to her desirability in the eyes of others; beyond that threat, and on a deeper level, I think, she is faced with a threat to her own identity. If she is truly to recover from such a loss, then, the language of the patriarchal beauty myth — "How can I make myself appear beautiful again?" won't adequately serve her. She also needs to ask, "How can I *feel* beautiful again? How can I feel that my body is still *my* body and therefore a body *I* can love?" If she is fortunate, she may be helped in her effort to achieve this psychic "recovery" by those who love her — and helped to no small degree. After all, a child's original knowledge of its body's beauty grows out of its security in knowing that its body is loved and cared for by another. And we may remember from our discussion of Burney's *Camilla*, how her family members and eventually her husband help the disfigured Eugenia recover her knowledge of herself as a whole person, rather than one whose "beautiful, good" spirit is forever trapped in an "ugly, bad" body: they do it, not by magically effecting some change in her aspect, but by loving her as a whole person. Ultimately, though, only the woman who has herself sustained the injury to her sense of her body's integrity (in the literal sense of the word — her body's wholeness) can recover the knowledge of herself as beautiful. In this chapter I want to tell two mastectomy narratives which reveal much about the nature of the psychic threat a woman undergoing this traumatic procedure feels. But even more important, I think, because more useful, are the suggestions these two narratives make about how a woman may find her way toward the psychic recovery of that same loss.

To define these true-life stories as *narratives* is to stress the way in which the writer in each case makes meaning out of the terror and confusion of her own experience, how she manages to discover a way of exerting some measure of control over an experience where, in an obvious sense, she has very little control. The meaning each writer makes of her experience will, I hope, be used by her readers in the same way that I have used the fictional narratives discussed in earlier chapters. The first narrative I will be telling here (second-hand) is Fanny Burney's, written in a letter to her sister; the second narrative is my own.

In 1811, when Fanny Burney was in her late fifties, living in Napoleonic France with her beloved husband the Count d'Arblay and their seventeen-year-old son, and working on her last novel, *The Wanderer*, a protest against tyrannies of various sorts, she underwent a traumatic experience of her own, with its own element of subjection to tyranny: the surgical excision, without anesthesia, of her right breast, to remove a large (and presumed to be cancerous) tumor. Some six months after the event, anticipating that news of her illness might soon reach family relations and friends back in England if it had not done so already, Burney began writing an account of the procedure in a letter home to her sister Esther, to assure the others of her "perfect recovery."[1] But Burney's letter does much more than provide such reassurance. To her beloved sister she promises to tell "the whole history" of the event, "certain that, from the moment you know any evil has befallen me your kind kind heart will be constantly anxious to learn its extent, & its circumstances, as well as its termination" (p. 128). Thus, though the contents of the letter are directed to be shared with the larger audience of family members and friends (with the exception of Burney's now elderly and always overly protective father), its form is that of intimate woman-to-woman discourse. From her sister Burney will withhold nothing; to her she will impart all the intimate details which one sister (with her "kind heart") would naturally wish to hear and the other to disclose. In this sense Burney's letter to her sister might be seen as the female counterpart to the man-to-man exchange in which the woman's body-parts are inventoried and appraised. The woman, however, talking about her own body, has a very different story to share with a member of her own sex.

As Julia Epstein has recently shown, Burney labored over her letter to Esther, revising it extensively (the letter was begun in March of 1812 but not finished till June — the surgery itself had been performed in September of the previous year), as she crafted the story of her own body's violation into a powerful work of art,[2] which has indeed a dramatic impact equalled by few moments in her fiction. We are justified in surmising that Burney's letter, though written to her sister Esther, was also written for posterity — that is, for us. And happily so, for its value is manifold. Over the years, Burney's account of her surgery has received considerable attention in medical circles, as one of the few in-depth descriptions, from a patient's point of view, of what it was like to experience a major surgical procedure before the benefits of anesthesia were available. (This is also only the third recorded account of the removal of a breast in a case of suspected cancer.) And Burney's narrative, with its harrowing description of the surgical procedure itself, is a powerful testimony to the human spirit's ability to endure the seemingly unendurable. But I think its value, as a social document, goes even further. Burney's mastectomy narrative is a powerful document in the history of the objectification of women's bodies by men in Western culture. And it is an even more powerful testimony to a woman's ability, even when thus subjected, and even when she is literally losing a part of her female body, to reassume possession of her body and her self. How Burney succeeds in "reframing" the events of her mastectomy — for she cannot undo the event itself — is a story that has much to teach us today. For we need, desperately, models for such reimagining. There are so many events in women's lives where our sense that we are the possessors of our own bodies is threatened — small events as well as large ones, but cumulative in their effects. No, we cannot control all that happens (perhaps not even most of what happens) to our bodies. Burney couldn't protect herself from the tumor that was growing in her breast; she couldn't protect herself from its surgical removal — and ultimately did not wish to do so. We, like she, cannot even protect ourselves from the sort of male gaze (and its ramifications in actions) that would deny our bodies their autonomy. But we can control how we respond to such experiences. And this is where Burney's mastectomy narrative, I think, is so valuable to us. It is an amazing story, and one which I want, for the most part, to let Burney tell us in her own words.

With a great novelist's sure sense of drama, Burney builds to her climax slowly. But she uses the opening section of her narrative, which describes in detail the events leading up to the surgery, to establish the sexual context in which the surgery itself will be placed. From the start we are in a world where the woman, who may or may not have something "wrong" with her, is exposed to the man's scrutiny and dependent on his judgment. She describes to Esther her discovery in the preceding year of a small pain in her breast, which continued to augment from week to week, until she was finally prevailed upon by "the most sympathising of Partners" to consult a surgeon and consent to an examination — an idea from which she "revolted," hoping that "by care & warmth," she might "make all succour unnecessary" (p. 128). It is customary today to ascribe the extreme anxiety felt by women in earlier centuries about exposing their bodies to examination by male physicians to a benighted prudishness. But consider for a moment the idea that those women were perhaps wiser than we. Perhaps they were more in touch with feelings which we, as "enlightened" women, feel we must censor. They knew that in exposing their bodies to the eye of the "good doctor," they might often be exposing themselves less to a knowing (and hence loving) eye than to a controlling and objec-

tifying one. Or maybe they understood, as we are beginning to discover again, that women at the least often pay a high price for the
"good doctor's" medical expertise. In any case, M. d'Arblay wisely
elicited the support of several of his wife's women friends over the
course of the next several months; and their persuasions, combined
with his own, finally induced her to overcome her repugnance and,
"most painfully & reluctantly," to consent to the examination.

No less an authority than M. Dubois, "the most celebrated surgeon of France" and accoucheur to the Empress, was called away
from his court attendance by Burney's devoted husband, for nothing "could slacken the ardour of M. d'A. to obtain the first advice"
(p. 128). Despite Burney's obvious gratitude for her husband's loving solicitude, what comes through in her narrative of the visit
from the great surgeon is the way in which the two men, with the
best will in the world, conspire to exclude Burney herself from the
truth-telling and decision-making process. When the great surgeon
has concluded his examination, he makes light of the problem to
Burney herself, simply giving her a prescription to follow for a
month — "but uttered so many charges to me to be tranquil, & suffer no uneasiness, that I could not but suspect there was room for
terrible inquietude." Burney is no fool: she knows exactly how to
read such pointed reassurances (who doesn't?). She continues
tellingly,

> My alarm was increased by the non-appearance of M. d'A. after
> his departure. They had remained together some time in the Book
> room, & M. d'A. did not return — till, unable to bear the suspence,
> I begged him to come back. He, also, sought then to tranquilize
> me — but in words only; his looks were shocking! his features,
> his whole face displayed the bitterest woe. I had not, therefore,
> much difficulty in telling myself what he endeavoured not to tell
> me — that a small operation would be necessary to avert evil con-
> sequences! — Ah, my dearest Esther, for this I felt no cour-
> age — my dread repugnance, for a thousand reasons *besides* the
> pain, almost shook all my faculties, &, for some time, I was rather
> confounded & stupified than affrighted.   (p. 129)

"A thousand reasons *besides* the pain." Terrible as that will be, the pain will indeed not be the worst of what Burney endures, as her ensuing narrative reveals. And much of what will make the experience of the surgery itself so terrifying is already being set in motion here, as the men make their preparations behind a closed door.

As the weeks pass, Burney feels the tumor growing and becoming increasingly painful: "I took, but vainly, my proscription, & every symptom grew more serious. At this time, M. de Narbonne spoke to M. d'A. of a Surgeon of great eminence, M. Larrey, who had cured a polonoise lady of his acquaintance of a similar malady; &, as my horror of an operation was insuperable, M. de N[arbonne] strongly recommended that I should have recourse to M. Larrey. I thankfully caught at any hope . . ." (p. 129). M. Larrey consents to take over the case, and a "new *regime*" is introduced, which for a time seems to produce good results: Burney feels better, goes out of the house, goes about her business. Happily for her, during this interval she is also getting to know her new physician, M. Larrey, and discovering him to be "one of the worthiest, most disinterested, & singularly excellent of men, endowed with real Genius in his profession, though with an ignorance of the World & its usages that induces a *naiveté* that leads those who do not see him thoroughly to think him not alone simple, but weak. They are mistaken . . ." (p. 130). Larrey, though delighted with Burney's improvement, insists on another consultation, with "le Docteur Ribe, the first anatomist, he said, in France, from his own fear lest he was under any delusion, from the excess of his desire to save me" (p. 130).

That last clause makes me like Larrey too. He recognizes his own attachment to Burney, a warm and empathetic woman as well as a famous novelist. He understands that his own desire to spare his patient the operation she so much dreads may be influencing his opinion of her condition, and calls for another opinion. The initial prognosis after this further examination seems again promising; but then once more the situation deteriorates. "The good M. Larrey, when he came to me next after the last of these trials, was quite thrown into a consternation, so changed he found all for the worse — 'Et qu'est il donc arrive?' he cried, & presently, sadly announced his hope[s] of dissolving the hardness were nearly extinguished" (p. 131). The former specialist, and then a third, are called in; a formal consultation ensues: "&, in fine, I was formally condemned to an operation by all Three" (p. 131).

Burney's own immediate response to this "sentence" is telling in the deep ambivalence it suggests about her feelings about her own body. On the one hand she expresses surprise — "I was as much astonished as disappointed — for the poor breast was no where discoloured, & not much larger than its healthy neighbor" (p. 131). The "not much larger" is puzzling in view of the testimony of the attending physician, appended to Burney's letter, which reports the tumor to be the size of a fist ("du Volume du poing," p. 141). But Burney's sense of surprise here may not be simply attributed to a natural impulse of denial. What she is really expressing here, I think, is her deep conviction of her body's essential innocence, or goodness, as that goodness is experienced on the most basic level — as a sense of bodily integrity: the "bad" breast does not seem fundamentally different to her from its counterpart, "its healthy neighbor." How can these important, powerful men be telling her that there is something terribly wrong in this sexual, life-giving part of herself? Burney's situation here is not unlike that of the "unfortunate Eugenia" in her fictional narrative *Camilla*. Like the disfigured Eugenia, she knows she hasn't done anything deserving of censure. And more deeply and securely than a young girl could, the happily married wife and mother knows her body's sexual value in a positive rather than a negative sense. For it resides not in her assurance of her virgin innocence but in the very fact of her sexual experience: has she not, at this very breast, suckled her own infant? (In a letter written three months after little Alex's birth, Burney tells of an infection transmitted to her breast from her infant's case of thrush, which caused her considerable pain.)[3] How, then, could something be "bad" in this life-sustaining part of her body?

As soon as Burney exclaims she is "astonished" to be told her breast is diseased, in the very next sentence, again like the fictional Eugenia, she expresses a deep sense of culpability — as if the tumor confirms her worst fears about her woman's body: "Yet I felt the evil to be deep, so deep, that I often thought if it could not be dissolved, it could only with life be extirpated" (p. 131). Just as one could see the initial response as denial of the disease, one could see this second, opposite response as an essentially healthy defense mechanism. Although present medical knowledge suggests that Burney's tumor was probably not malignant — since had it been so, given its large size, it probably would have already metastasized and Burney would not have lived in relatively good health for another thirty years after her surgery — *she* would nevertheless need to convince herself that "the evil" inside her was indeed life-threatening if she were to get through the ordeal ahead of her. Her terminology here, however, that the evil could only be extirpated *with life*, suggests to me rather that she is feeling what even an essentially psychologically healthy woman feels in such a situation: that she — in her whole being — must be bad if this evil thing is inside her. Or rather, what she feels is the contradiction between the two states: on the one hand, in this most fundamental aspect of her nature, she knows she is good; on the other hand, the fact of the tumor's existence inside her "proves" she is bad.

What emerges from the turmoil of her ambivalent responses, though, is a determination to see the thing through, and she regains her self-possession in a touching expression of her confidence in the surgeon-executioner who is, after all, also her ally in the battle for her life. And this is where the friendship that has developed between Burney and Larrey in the intervening period is so critical: Burney's sense of allegiance with Larrey seems to me crucial here. "I called up," she says, "all the reason I possessed, or could assume, & told them — that if they saw no other alternative, I would not resist their opinion & experience: — the good Dr. Larrey, who, during his long attendance had conceived for me the warmest friendship, had now tears in his Eyes; from my dread he had expected resistance. He proposed again calling in M. Dubois [the first consultant]. No, I told him, if I could not by himself be saved, I had no sort of hope elsewhere, &, if it must be, what I wanted in courage should be supplied by Confidence" (p. 131). Finally, after yet another examination, the doctors once more consult behind closed doors:

> I left them — what an half hour I passed alone! — M. d'A. was at his office. Dr. Larrey then came to summon me. He did not speak, but looked very like my dear Brother James, to whom he has a personal resemblance that has struck M. d'A. as well as myself. I came back, & took my seat, with what calmness I was able. All were silent, & Dr. Larrey, I saw, hid himself nearly behind my Sofa. My heart beat fast: I saw all hope was over. I called upon them to speak. M. Dubois then, after a long & unintelligible harangue, from his own disturbance, pronounced my doom. I now saw it was inevitable, and abstained from any further effort. They received my formal consent, & retired to fix a day. *(p. 132)*

We can see Burney here gathering her resources, finding the means by which she will best be able to deal with the upcoming trauma. Not only does she accept the inevitable with the best grace she can muster, but she does all she can to domesticate and demystify her powerful male executioners. Larrey is to be the man, and so it is important for her at this moment to notice his resemblance to a beloved brother, and also to notice that Larrey himself (in an exaggerated mime of her own trepidation) is, at least in her view, nearly hiding himself behind the couch. It *helps* to discover that the executioner also has human feelings, that it gives him pain to inflict pain on us.

Burney does a valiant job of trying, in advance, to maintain some control over the terrible assault that is about to take place on her body. But it is difficult. Indeed, while in many ways these doctors come across as more enlightened and caring than many of their counterparts today, they still find ways of making the experience one which cannot but feel disempowering and humiliating to her. The doctors — and it is important that it is the less sympathetic but most highly positioned M. Dubois who takes charge here — assume knowing ahead of time exactly when the operation is to occur will only heighten her anxiety (or, perhaps more accurately, they are determined to retain control over the proceedings themselves). Despite Burney's pleadings, they will "not suffer me to know the time myself over night; I obtained with difficulty a promise of 4 hours warning, which were essential to me for sundry regulations" (p. 133). Nor is she informed what supplies will be necessary. (The surgery is to be performed in her own home.) "All that to *me* was owned, as wanting, was an arm Chair & some Towels" (p. 133) — while meanwhile, unknown to her, various other supplies, compresses, bandages, wooden "charpie" (splints?), were being gathered and hidden away in a closet.

Burney's handling of "the most sympathising of Partners" is interesting here. Initially M. d'A. is among the party of deliberating men; after the decision is made, however, he is increasingly shut out from the masculine conclave. And indeed, he is excluded at Burney's own express desire. (Her wish is supported by all the attending physicians but the humane Larrey himself.) M. d'A. is not to be present during the surgery itself; in fact he is not even to be told it is taking place until it is all over. Unknown to him, Burney makes out her will — which fact she confesses to her sister she still to this day has not told him, fearing that until he is fully assured of her recovery "it might still affect him" (p. 133). She now turns the focus of her energies to "assum[ing] the best spirits in my power, *to meet the coming blow*; — & support my too sympathising Partner" (p. 133). There is a kind of turning of the tables on M. d'A. here — a familiar maneuver on the part of two mutually protective members of a marriage when the health of one is threatened. Now *he* is the one from whom frightening truths must be hidden and contrived to be kept out of the way! Or, protecting her husband, keeping him even less informed than she is, enables Burney to assert some measure of control; it gives her someone else to worry about besides herself.

Then, as she is dressing herself one morning, with only two hours' notice instead of the promised four, she receives a letter from Larrey:

to acquaint me that at 10 o'clock he should be with me, properly accompanied, & to exhort me to rely as much upon his sensibility & his prudence, as upon his dexterity & his experience; he charged to secure the absence of M. d'A. . . . Judge, my Esther, if I read this [bulletin from the surgeon] unmoved! — yet I had to disguise my sensations & intentions from M. d'A! — Dr. Aumont, the Messenger & terrible Herald, was in waiting; M. d'A. stood by my bed side; I affected to be long reading the Note, to gain time for forming some plan, & such was my terror of involving M. d'A. in the unavailing wretchedness of witnessing what I must go through, that it conquered every other, & gave me the force to act as if I were directing some third person. *(p. 135)*

She sends her son privately to M. d'A.'s chief at the bureau where he is employed, telling him "*the moment was come,*" and asking him to summon her husband to the office and to keep him there on the pretext of some urgent business until all is over. When I first read this passage I could not understand why Burney would banish a truly loving and sympathetic mate from a position if not at her side at least in the house, where he might be close by at such a terrible time. Her letter includes a postscript to the dear English friends from M. d'A. which gives me my answer:

No! No my dearest & ever more dear friends, I shall not make a fruitless attempt. No language could convey what I felt in the deadly course of those seven hours. Nevertheless, every one *of you, my dearest dearest friends*, can guess, must even know it. Alexandre [their son] had no less feeling, but showed more fortitude. He, perhaps, will be more able to describe to you, nearly at least, the torturing state of my poor heart & soul. Besides, I must own, to you, that these details which were, till just now, quite unknown to me, have almost killed me, & I am only able to thank God that this more than half Angel has had the sublime courage to deny herself the comfort I might have offered her, to spare me, not the sharing of her excruciating pains, that was impossible, but the witnessing so terrific a scene, & perhaps the remorse to have rendered it more tragic. For I don't flatter myself I could have got through it — I must confess it. *(pp. 140–41)*

Burney knew her husband. And she also knew herself, knew that setting herself the task of protecting *him* would help her, as she says, to think of herself as a third person — as it were, a character in one of her own fictions whose responses she can manipulate, thus perhaps gaining a necessary measure of distance from what will be happening to her body.

There is a knock at the door. What follows reads like one of the emotionally taut seduction scenes from Richardson's *Clarissa*:

I rang for my Maid & Nurses, — but before I could speak to them, my room, without previous message, was entered by 7 Men in black, Dr. Larry [*sic*], M. Dubois, Dr. Moreau, Dr. Aumont, Dr. Ribe, & a pupil of Dr. Larry, & another of M. Dubois. I was now awakened from my stupor — & by a sort of indignation — Why so many? & without leave? — But I could not utter a syllable. M. Dubois acted as Commander in Chief. Dr. Larry kept out of sight; M. Dubois ordered a Bed stead into the middle of the room. Astonished, I turned to Dr. Larry, who had promised that an Arm Chair would suffice; but he hung his head, & would not look at me. Two *old mattrasses* M. Dubois then demanded, & an old Sheet. I now began to tremble violently, more with distaste & horrour of the preparations even than of the pain. These arranged to his liking, he desired me to mount the Bed stead. I stood suspended, for a moment, whether I should not abruptly escape — I looked at the door, the windows — I felt desperate — but it was only for a moment, my reason then took the command, & my fears & feelings struggled vainly against it. I called to my maid — she was crying, & the two Nurses stood, transfixed, at the door. Let those women all go! cried M. Dubois. This order recovered me my Voice — No, I cried, let them stay! *qu'elles restent!* This occasioned a little dispute, that re-animated me — The maid, however, & one of the nurses ran off — I charged the other to approach, & she obeyed. M. Dubois now tried to issue his commands *en militaire*, but I resisted all that were resistable — I was compelled, however, to submit to taking off my long robe de Chambre, which I had meant to retain — Ah, then, how did I think of my Sisters! — not one, at so dreadful an instant, at hand,

to protect — adjust — guard me — I regretted that I had refused
Me de Mainsonneuve — Me Chastel — no one upon whom I
could rely — my departed Angel! — how did I think of her! [this
last must be a reference to her most loved, deceased sister, Susan-
nah] — how did I long — long for my Esther — my Charlotte! —

(pp. 136–37)

The ordeal, as Burney stages it for us, begins with the confronta-
tion between the militaristic man and the woman who is determined to preserve what she can of her integrity as a human being — knowing that only by doing so can she endure the assault on
the integrity of her body. The substitution of the bedstead for the
promised armchair is no small setback to her effort here — as Larrey
would have surely realized in making the promise in the first place.
Lying prone on the bed she becomes, of course, all the more victim-
ized: the drama becomes all the more staged as a rape scene. Interestingly, what enables Burney to regain her composure, even while
submitting with grace to the inevitable, is her insistence, against the
stern doctor's command, on retaining her women by her side. No
sooner does the despotic M. Dubois command that her serving
women, cowering by the door, be sent away, than she insists that
they remain: "[His] order recovered me my Voice — No, I cried,
let them stay!" The female presence, by helping her to desexualize
the experience, is perhaps comforting in a way that her husband's
might not have been.

Having thus "re-animated" herself, Burney is able to take what
I think is the crucial action in her transformation of the event — an
act of sympathetic imagination.

My distress was, I suppose, apparent, though not my Wishes, for
M. Dubois himself now softened, & spoke soothingly. Can *You*,
I cried, feel for an operation that, to *You*, must seem so trivial? — Trivial? he repeated — taking up a bit of paper, which he tore,
unconsciously, into a million of pieces, *oui — c'est peu de chose —
mais —* ' he stammered, & could not go on. No one else attempted
to speak, but I was softened myself, when I saw even M. Dubois
grow agitated, while Dr. Larry kept always aloof, yet a glance
shewed me he was pale as ashes.

How wonderful of Burney, at such a moment, to notice the great surgeon unconsciously, in his anxiety for her, tearing to bits a piece of paper! And, from her point of view, how salutary! For it enables her to recognize more fully than she has yet done, the ultimate threat which hangs over her — a threat much larger than that posed by the surgery itself: "I knew not, positively, then, the immediate danger, but every thing convinced me danger was hovering about me, & that this experiment could alone save me from its jaws" (pp. 137–38). Because she has been able to see them as human beings, with feelings like her own, Burney is able to suddenly see the men who threaten violation as the agents of her salvation. And having seen them thus, she can then take it upon herself to mount "unbidden, the Bed stead" (138). Immediately a cambric handkerchief is placed over her face:

> It was transparent, however, & I saw, through it, that the Bed stead was instantly surrounded by the 7 men & my nurse. I refused to be held; but when, Bright through the cambric, I saw the glitter of polished Steel — I closed my Eyes. I would not trust to convulsive fear the sight of the terrible incision. A silence the most profound ensued, which lasted for some minutes, during which, I imagine, they took their orders by signs, & made their examination — Oh what a horrible suspension! — I did not breathe — & M. Dubois tried vainly to find any pulse. This pause, at length was broken by Dr. Larry, who in a voice of solemn melancholy, said, 'Qui me tiendra ce sein?' ["Who will hold this breast for me?"]
>
> No one answered; at least not verbally; but this aroused me from my passively submissive state, for I feared they imagined the whole breast infected — feared it too justly — for, again through the Cambric, I saw the hand of M. Dubois held up, while his fore finger first described a straight line from top to bottom of the breast, secondly a Cross, & thirdly a Circle; intimating that the WHOLE was to be taken off.

I find it appalling, reading this, to realize that Burney must have gone into the surgery expecting what we would call a lumpectomy will be performed, and only now realizes her whole breast is to be removed. (M. Dubois' directions imply that Larrey himself, as the mere surgeon in this case, rather than chief director of the operation, is himself only following orders.) My shock aside, the point is that Burney obviously has not been informed, and it is her shock of disempowerment that galvanizes her into action. Her words, at this moment, are for me, the most moving in the entire narrative:

> Excited by this idea, I started up, threw off my veil, &, in answer to the demand "Qui me tiendra ce sein?" cried "C'est moi, Monsieur!" & I held my hand under it, & explained the nature of my sufferings, which all sprang from one point, though they darted into every part. I was heard attentively, but in utter silence, & M. Dubois then re-placed me as before, &, as before, spread my veil over my face. How vain, alas, my representation! — immediately again I saw the fatal finger describe the Cross — & the circle — Hopeless, then, desperate, & self-given up, I closed once more my Eyes, relinquishing all watching, all resistance, all interference, & sadly resolute to be wholly resigned.
>
> My dearest Esther, — & all my dears to whom she communicates this doleful ditty, will rejoice to hear that this resolution once taken, was firmly adhered to, in defiance of a terror that surpasses all description, & the most torturing pain.   (p. 138)

Burney's account of the twenty minutes (!) of cutting and scraping and finally the dressing of the wound is truly harrowing. But the truly important part of the narrative is the part I have just quoted, which deals with the prelude to the surgery itself; for it is here that Burney struggles to come to terms with the ordeal she is about to experience; and here is her victory. Although Burney is denied her plea that she may be the one to hold her own breast during the surgery — since M. Dubois has decreed that there will be no remaining part of the breast which might be so held — symbolically if not literally I think Burney does indeed "hold her own breast" through her ordeal. She does it by holding on to, or reclaiming, herself — both in body and in spirit. She does it by refusing simply to play out her assigned part in the drama of the violated woman. She insists on her own right to alter the script where she can, and where she cannot, to perform her role with dignity and without any prompting — and that in itself is to redefine the role. For the woman who gets onto the bed herself is the woman who is about to have a life-saving surgical operation performed on her body, not the helpless victim of a rape. Moreover, to my mind, perhaps the most important aspect of Burney's revision of the assigned script is her ability to discover the humanity of her male "assailants," understanding that they too belong to a social world which none of them has created, and that if they are her surgeons, they are also her protectors — not simply because they are in truth trying to save her life, but because they are human beings with feelings of their own — or rather the second insight makes possible the first.

Burney's ability to identify with her doctors, particularly with Larrey, and *his* equally important ability to break through *his* professional role and identify with *her*, comes through strongly at the very end of the narrative: "However, I bore it with all the courage I could exert, & never moved, nor stopt them, nor resisted, nor remonstrated, nor spoke — except once or twice, during the dressings, to say, 'Ah Messieurs! que je vous plains! — ' ['Oh, good sirs, I beg you — '] for indeed I was sensible to the feeling concern with which they all saw what I endured, though my speech was principally — *very* principally meant for Dr. Larry. Except this, I uttered not a syllable . . ." (p. 140).

At the very end, when she is carried back to her own bed, Burney says, "This removal made me open my Eyes — & I then saw my good Dr. Larry, pale nearly as myself, his face streaked with blood, & its expression depicting grief, apprehension, & almost horror. When I was in bed, — my poor M. d'Arblay — who ought to write you himself his own history of this Morning — was called to me — & afterwards our Alex" (p. 140).

Feeling so strongly that the kind of mutual sympathy that existed between Larrey and Burney, a male physician (particularly a surgeon) and a female patient, is something rare and wonderful in any age, I was surprised recently to read a very different account of this same relationship in a contemporary work by a practicing surgeon, Dr. Richard Selzer. In the preface to a memoir on his own experiences both as a patient and a surgeon, *Raising the Dead*,⁴ Selzer uses the Burney-Larrey relationship as a cautionary tale. Describing the friendship that developed between Larrey and Burney before the surgery, Selzer comments, "This was to the great benefit of Fanny, but it may have cost Larrey, who was seduced by his charming and vivacious patient into stripping off the protective carapace that is necessary to any man whose work it is to lay open the bodies of his fellow human beings." But how has the "seduction" harmed her surgeon? It hasn't *prevented* him from getting his job done; in fact, by providing the surgeon with an unmoving object, rather than a resistant, writhing one, on which to perform his delicate work, the friendship probably helped rather than hindered the surgeon's action. But it also exposed the male doctor to his feelings; he couldn't just walk away from the ordeal when it was over, untouched by it. Burney describes Larrey's aspect, after the completion of the surgery, in a way that underlines the fact that they have been through something *together*: he is "pale *nearly as myself*" (my italics) and "his face [is] streaked with blood" (p. 140) — *her* blood. Yes, in a sense, Larrey has made it harder for himself; but by allowing Burney to see his own suffering (and, as I have suggested, it is to Burney's credit that she *can* see that) this surgeon has made an agonizing ordeal more bearable for his patient — the real sufferer here. My definition of a *good* doctor, not a *bad* one! Significantly, Selzer misplaces and misreads Burney's "que je vous plains!" placing it *before* Larrey makes the incision, as if it were a plea for him to refrain, instead of coming, as she tells us it did, during the bandaging, when the cutting is all over, and being (as she makes clear) as much a comment on her sympathy for her physicians as a plea for mercy. Selzer allows that we might possibly "forgive" Fanny for her "self-indulgence" on this occasion.

But really, I shouldn't be surprised. Narratives like Selzer's will continue to be written, for the ideal of male-female relations they set forth (an ideal, obviously not limited to the relations between doctors and patients) has endured for a long time and does not seem

likely to die out. It is Burney's story that is the truly surprising —
and important — one, the one for us to remember and to make use
of in our own lives. Her "mastectomy narrative" is a triumph of
courage: the courage to endure an almost unthinkable degree of
physical pain; and the courage to transform a story of a woman's disempowerment into a story not so much of her empowerment —
though there is that — but of her humanity in the largest sense.

Burney's offer to hold her own breast during the surgery —
"c'est moi qui tiendra ce sein" — and the physical gesture she makes
to reenforce that offer, actually taking the breast in her hand are
complex in their meaning. Her gesture is one of compliance or sac-
rifice: she will give this up. It is a gesture of defiance: if she holds
onto her breast then they cannot take it (all) away. More importantly, still, it is a gesture which expresses her need to participate in
the procedure about to take place: if she can take an active role in
what is happening to her body, she can and will save herself. And
perhaps on an even deeper, more primitive level, it is an affirmation
of self-esteem, in which an "ugly," offending, sexual part of her
body is converted, by her own touch, into a beautiful, loved part.
Like a more grown-up version of Drabble's Sarah, Burney is affirming the essential virtue — the strength as well as the goodness — of her body by hugging her own body in her own arms. And
that is the action we need most to enable ourselves to perform.

Two years ago (like Burney, I've taken time to compose my narrative), I agreed to undergo a mastectomy in order to save my life.
And, as she was, I was totally unprepared to hear the full "sentence"
when it came. Not that anyone misled me about the extent of the
procedure beforehand, nor (what may have been more likely in
Burney's case) allowed me to mislead myself. It's rather that mammography makes it possible to detect the presence of malignancy
before there is any lump a woman can feel in her breast. Mammography provides a great advantage, obviously, from a medical point
of view: early intervention made me one of the lucky ones, a sur-

vivor. But this medical advance can also mean, as it did in my case, that the sentence of "mastectomy" can come to the woman as a total shock.

Some tiny "suspicious" dots had shown up on my routine mammogram. It was explained to me that occasionally such dots (themselves marks of calcification) were indicators of the presence of malignancy: I would need a biopsy. Upsetting, but O.K., I thought. I can deal with this, and I rapidly constructed (the way one does) a "worst case scenario" in my mind: the "bad" part, if it was there, would be taken away. There couldn't be very much, for the dots were so tiny I couldn't even see them until they showed me an enlargement of the X-ray. Was this wishful thinking? I don't know. I do know it's very hard for the mind to process something one has no awareness of in one's body.

First would come the biopsy. That shouldn't be too bad, I thought. In the radiology department, with the aid of an X-ray, a line of dye would be injected into the exact spot where the dots were within the breast tissue. Then up to surgery, where, following the path of the dye, the surgeon would know just where to remove the tissue for the biopsy.

But it was bad. The position I was asked to assume, with my breast squeezed between two sheets of metal, like for a mammogram only much worse, was one I found intolerably painful. I told the attendant I didn't think I could hold that position for the five minutes or so it would take to inject the dye. She agreed to a different position, not pleasant but bearable. The radiologist then entered, followed by another man — a colleague? a student? I couldn't see either one of them because they were standing in back of me, as I was gripped by the vice. The radiologist explained to the person accompanying him that they would not be doing the procedure in the usual way "because the patient didn't like it," but he thought the results would be satisfactory. They continued talking to each other, as one demonstrated what he was doing; no one said anything to me.

And then that part was over. I knew how Burney felt when the seven men crowded around her as she lay with the cambric cloth over her face. And indeed the pain was the least of it. I'd gotten my first taste of what I would be up against. But I didn't realize that then; I assumed the worst was over. The biopsy itself I have no recollection of, perhaps because what had happened in the radiologist's office felt so humiliating. I hoped that would be the end of it, and waited — anxiously, of course — for the visit with the surgeon four or five days later.

It did not occur to me to ask a friend to accompany me to the surgeon's office. The doctor examined me, and then we sat down in his office. He explained that, yes, there was evidence of malignancy, but the cancerous cells were contained within the ducts and that was good. The prognosis was excellent. "You're telling me I'll need surgery, then," I said. What exactly would they do? And he said "a mastectomy." Perhaps I should have been prepared to hear that sentence; perhaps I was "defended" against it. (Perhaps Burney should have known it was all going to be taken off too.) But I wasn't. I remember screaming over and over in my disbelief as I sat in the doctor's office, feeling terribly alone. After a few minutes, the doctor explained, very kindly, that the cells were "multi-focal," diffuse throughout the specimen tissue. There was no way of knowing where the border might be; so to be sure, they would have to take it all. I remember feeling that this couldn't possibly be really happening. He couldn't really be telling me I had to lose a breast when I had no sense of anything at all being wrong. And I remember thinking, "How will I be able to take care of my daughter in this? How will I protect her?"

After some time — days or weeks I'm not sure — I got myself to believe it was going to happen, and like Burney I began to find ways of preparing myself. But, although intellectually I understood that what was about to happen to me was a life-saving action, I don't think I could ever *experience* it in those terms. After all, there was nothing there that I could feel; I felt in every sense perfectly well. How could there be something that "bad" inside my body? It didn't feel consoling to be told either by doctors or by other women that

I was "lucky." Two years later, I still find myself reliving, from time to time, that moment of shock in the doctor's office, and my screams — like those of a terrified animal. I guess I still need to relive it, to take it in.

Of course, in many ways my experience was so much easier than Burney's — and not simply because it was virtually free of any extreme physical pain. I had a number of supports she missed, or for complicated reasons did not permit herself to receive. I asked my closest woman friend to come with me for the two important visits to surgeons before the operation, not for advice but to be there for me. I didn't want to be taken by surprise all by myself again; and I knew I wouldn't be able to hear everything they said (which certainly proved to be the case). Toni took some notes, asked a few questions: mainly she was just there. And there, afterwards, to stand on the street-corner with me, "decompressing." I said I thought the pictures we'd seen of the reconstructed breasts looked terrible; she thought they weren't all that bad: we discussed it. Then, several weeks later, my own much-loved sister came to be with me at the time of the surgery and stayed for several days thereafter — and that made a great difference. I am also blessed in having two beloved mother figures in my life now; both of them called me every day in the week following the surgery and frequently in the days and months thereafter. And in a different way it helped to have a twelve-year-old daughter who I knew was going to be more scared than I was, and who needed to know that her mother was going to be all right. Since that was an assurance I could give her honestly, that helped too. I told her I was having the operation so I would *not* get sick, so something bad would *not* happen. And telling her that made me realize it was true: the little abnormal cells in the duct tissue weren't doing me a bit of harm now. It was only if they escaped from the duct, and then from the breast altogether, getting into other parts of my body where they could damage other vulnerable life-supporting organs that I would become sick; only if we let that happen, would it be bad. I was fine now, and I was going to stay that way. That made sense to both of us. (Somehow this analysis felt different from convincing myself that I was "lucky." There didn't seem to be anything fortunate at all about what was about to happen, but I did know that I wanted and needed to maintain the good health I have.) I guess my daughter was for me what Burney's husband was for her—someone *I* needed to protect. And I was more fortunate than Burney in having an adult male friend who could be there to take care of me rather than needing to be taken care of himself. And probably that made the biggest difference of all.

Also I had my own M. Larrey—not in my case the surgeon, but my own physician. When I was still in a state of shock, sitting in the surgeon's office that first afternoon, one of us suggested we inform Dr. Tesher of the results of the biopsy—so we phoned him. Dr. T. asked me if I'd like to stop by his office and I thought perhaps I would. This was a doctor whom I'd known well for four years and liked enormously, though our relationship had never really been tested: my health had never before been in serious jeopardy. I walked the ten blocks to his office in a daze, and cried tears (instead of screams) while he put his arms around me. He shared the distress *with* me: it didn't bowl him over, but he let me know he hadn't expected this outcome either, and wondered out loud whether he ought to have. A good doctor, like Larrey. He reassured me that I would get through it, that he'd be there to help me; and he told me a little about breast reconstruction, saying it could be begun (if I wanted) at the same time as the mastectomy itself.

But of course, having all that love and support around me could not do everything. I don't mean that it couldn't insulate me from suffering: of course it couldn't do that. I mean it couldn't insulate me from the sort of horrible surprises and humiliations I had already gotten a taste of in the radiologist's office, and which Burney experienced at more than one point—moments at which one's sense of having some measure of control over, or participation in, what is happening to one's body, is suddenly wrested away, and a life-saving surgical procedure becomes instead a nightmare experience of sexual exposure and violation. In the week prior to my surgery, a friend had given me Betty Rollins's powerful and honest account of her mastectomy experience, *First You Cry*. I had been terrified by Rollins's vivid description of the moment when she finally got up the courage, about a month after her surgery, to look at the incision itself: "On the left half of my chest, where a breast had been, was a flat, lumpy surface like the ground, covered with, instead of dirt, skin. Across the surface, a long, horizontal, red, puffy welt meandered crazily from the center of my chest, where a cleavage once was, to the other side, under the arm, and around toward the back.

And alongside this little Hiroshima of the torso, on the unbombed half, grotesque by contrast, lay a right breast, pretty and whole as a healthy baby."[5]

We react variously to physical mutilation; but I knew I was like Rollins and would react as she had. Surreptitious glances in my childhood at the victims of burns and skin infections in my father's medical textbooks had been enough to convince me that medicine was not the profession for me, after all. When, as a full grown adult, I slammed a car door on the end of my thumb, it had taken me at least a week to be able to look at my squashed (but still intact) finger. How was I ever going to be able to deal with this injury to my body? It went deeper, of course, than the feeling of squeamishness about physical injury. A part of the body that has to be destroyed, in Rollins's metaphor a fertile country turned by an act of cataclysmic violence into barren, war-scarred earth, must have been a bad place to begin with. That she should see her remaining, intact breast at this moment not in sexual terms but as the emblem of an infant's innocence and vulnerability made sense to me: the untouched, "good" breast is a terrible reminder of the intact, loved infant she feels she once was but can never be again. Rollins's description here is so powerful because it speaks to the intensity of the feelings we have about our body's wholeness — the very proof of our essential goodness. To lose a part of our body is to lose something more than a physical part of oneself: it threatens our essential sense of selfhood.

Particularly a sexual part. And particularly, for me, a sexual part that never got to perform its proper function — that of nursing a baby. (My daughter, Ruth, is an adopted child.) I knew that losing a breast, for me, would feel devastating not simply because a breast is the most visible symbol of a woman's femininity — and hence of her attractiveness to men. It would feel devastating to me because it would be losing the thing itself — the breast as the woman's nurturing organ. It would be just one more "proof" that, from a reproductive point of view, my body had failed me. It hadn't produced the baby when I'd wanted one: now this other part of my woman's body was betraying me as well, another proof of my defectiveness. Of course I knew that this complex of feelings wasn't rational — the same feelings expressed in that first inarticulate scream of disbelief in the doctor's office but now realized more fully and clearly as I read Rollins's description of seeing the "bombed" place where her breast had been. I knew that just because a woman has lost a breast doesn't mean she can never feel whole again; I certainly knew intellectually, just as Burney had, that the tiny misshaped cells multiplying inside my breast ducts were not signs of any psychic or sexual failing inside me. But I also knew, more intensely for reading Rollins's account, how real these feelings were — real and therefore to be respected. I felt terrified reading Rollins's account of her mastectomy — terrified and also enlightened. Losing a breast, as Rollins makes brutally clear in her book, *First You Cry*, is a devastating narcissistic injury for a woman — not one which can't be survived, but one which demands grieving, hard work, and in the end, somehow, a restoration of one's self esteem.

Reading Rollins's narrative was useful to me in another way as well. It made me realize I would need to think carefully about when and under what circumstances I wanted to take that first look at myself. I knew that I would want to do what I could to place the shock (if it was to be one) in a setting that would feel most reassuring to me. And it was reassuring to think I could choose when and how to take that first look: here was a piece of it I could control. (I would like to think Rollins would agree with me about the subjective basis of her description here. Perhaps if someone had been there who loved her, and loved her body, when she first looked at herself after the surgery, the wound might have looked very different to her.) I was very sure that I did not want to see my body while I was still in the hospital (in my case, a stay of a mere day and a half). And I did not do so. But the morning after the surgery a young assistant to my surgeon came into my room, when I was still feeling fairly out of it, with a younger female assistant in tow. "I'm one of your surgeon's elves," he said brightly. "I'll just be changing your dressing and taking a look at things." I carefully averted my face while he unwrapped the dressing. Then, as the two of them stood over me, he began pointing out to his apprentice the various features of what the two of them were looking at. "Here is the drain," he said, "and these are the skin flaps." He prodded around a bit, wrapped me up again, and said a cheerful goodbye. The student nodded to me, smiled, and the two of them left the room.

What are skin flaps, I wondered. Then suddenly I remembered the term from the reading I had done in a medical self-help book in the previous week. The "skin flaps" are the small pieces of skin which remain when all the breast tissue and the skin immediately over the site of the tumor had been removed; the "skin flaps" were simply all that remained of what had been my left breast. I think that the feelings of mixed humiliation and indignation I experienced in those few moments were the most painful ones in the whole experience for me. I felt as though I had tried to protect myself and not been able to do so, that my body was not even a part of me any more: it belonged to the two doctors and their world of medical know-how. And, interestingly, I do not think the fact that the assistant in this case was a woman made a bit of difference in my sense of violation: they might just as well both have been women. In terms of the dynamic of the "male gaze" and its reduction of the woman's body to a spectacle for the viewer to make use of as he (or she) chooses, the sex of the viewer does not make any difference. A woman can do to another woman's body what men have traditionally done to women's bodies just as well.

When the dressing came off for good, to be replaced by a small bandage, about four days later in the surgeon's office, I knew I was not yet ready to look at the wound myself. But I wanted very much for the man who loved me and had been caring for me to be there and for *him* to see it. Alan stood on the other side of the doctor while the dressing was being changed, and while I cried he remained calm. He looked at what I could not bring myself to look at myself, and I looked at his face. What I saw was that he looked at my body as he always had looked at it — curiously, interestedly, with the face of love. I realize, thinking back about my need to have Alan there to see the wound before I did, that I must have felt very secure about his response. Not in the sense that his view, as a man's, would supersede my own, but that he would love my body now because he always had loved it before. Which is really to say that what I felt secure about was his love for me. When he said later that it looked rather neat and tidy, a slightly curved shape with a thin line crossing the surface horizontally, I knew that eventually I would be able to see it that way too — if not quite yet.

Then, that same afternoon, alone and by pre-arrangement — I had planned everything out very carefully, knowing what would be best for me — I went from the surgeon's office to Dr. Tesher's office. Dr. T. didn't make light of my squeamishness. Before we went into his examining room he told me a story about how he himself, an avid skier, had had a bad skiing accident several years ago, as a result of which he had lost much of the use of his left arm. (A loss, incidentally, I'd never noticed.) And even though he was a physician who had himself performed surgery many times, he had not found it easy, he told me, to look at his mutilated arm that first time. His telling me this story at that moment helped me to do another thing that Burney found a way to do for herself — to see the male doctor who is in charge of her woman's body as a person with a vulnerable body of his own, and with his own fears about mutilation. Then we went into the examining room, Dr. T. undid my dressing, put on his glasses, looked carefully at the incision, commented on just where the suture lines went, and told me that the surgeon had done a good clean job. Finally I felt ready to look myself. And they were right; it really did not look so terrible, not nearly as bad as the description in the Betty Rollins book had led me to expect. Her surgery, for one thing, had been performed more than fifteen years earlier; perhaps changes in surgical procedure had made it possible to achieve a smoother, less mutilated look in the skin surface now. Also, since at the same time my mastectomy was performed I had undergone the initial stage of breast reconstruction (a technique not yet developed in 1975), the surface *I* saw was slightly convex rather than one slightly concave; and that small difference, I suspect, made a rather large difference in how our eyes, respectively, processed what we saw. The loss was still very real, but I did not have to convert, in that single instant, a positive space into a negative one. But most important, I feel sure, was the way the experience was framed for me by the presence of two men who knew me and cared for me in different ways, but whom I knew I could count on to look at me through eyes of love, and thus help me to know my body again myself as something lovable. I might speculate as to why I needed so much to see my body after the surgery first through those other, loving eyes. The analogy here, I suspect, is with the way a child's knowledge of itself as beautiful is predicated on the certainty of the mother's unfailing love — a love which makes it impossible for the mother to see her child's body as anything other than beautiful. Perhaps at a time when my self-esteem was inevitably called into question, and when my body felt both very vulnerable and very new, I had to reexperience myself as I would have been seen at the very beginning by a loving mother *before* I could trust to my own perception. But having assured myself of that "primary" love, when I looked at my body myself I was able to regain my own sense of my body as something beautiful, and thus to regain my sense of myself.

The rest of it, though, I had to do myself — the harder part. I had to be able, like Burney, to take my own breast (or, like Drabble's Sarah, my own body) in my own hand — and still know it as my body, still love it. But I don't think that I could have taken that next step without Alan being there to help me with the first one.

I'm afraid that without him I might have seen something much more like what Betty Rollins saw. And still, I knew it would be hard: for the truth was, my body was different now, and I would need time — I have needed time — to get to know this new body, to incorporate this new, unfamiliar piece into the old familiar whole.

It has taken me just about two years, or up till the time of the present writing. The physical recovery from the initial surgery, by contrast, took very little time at all: from the point of view of the body-organism as a whole, a breast is an add-on. I was up and feeling perfectly able to function in most ways within a matter of days. That was important to my daughter because it was a sign that I really was alright: we could both exult in the fact that I was "in such good shape" that my surgeon dismissed me from the hospital after just a day and a half. (I was certainly anxious to avoid any more encounters with those elves!) But in fact my body is not the same. Whether or not I had decided to undergo breast reconstruction, the recovery process would still have involved getting to know a new body. Since I had decided to undergo that process, what I needed to get to know and eventually to accept as a part of myself was a body that was not only different but, for a period of about a year and a half, changing. The whole process, in fact, particularly the initial six weeks during which the implant is gradually being inflated as the "skin flaps" must stretch to make room for the balloon growing inside them, had for me some of the feeling of the original growth of the breasts at puberty, when one watches with mingled feelings the shape of one's body change. The difference of course, is that while puberty's changes prepare the woman's body for childbearing, I can't pretend that this new imitation breast has any function to perform — other than to mimic the shape of its companion on the other side. "Reconstruction" might be considered a euphemism, since what one ends up with is obviously not a newly constructed breast, nor something that feels like one's other breast *from the inside*. The goal is to create something that will look, *from the outside*, as much as possible like the original breast. And yet, for me at least, my new, reconstructed breast, serves a function that goes beyond that of fooling others about what's underneath my clothing or perhaps of helping me to fool myself. In a way that's hard to explain but very real, it helps me regain a sense of my body's intactness. Perhaps that sense is something I could have come to without undergoing breast reconstruction. What I do feel strongly is that, however one achieves it, it is enormously important that a woman who has lost a breast, without denying the reality of that loss, still be able, at whatever time is the right time for her — and for me that's just about now, two years after the event — to say to herself, "This body is my body — different, but still my body."

Recent research on the "phantom limb" phenomenon, in which patients who have lost a limb continue to report sensations (sometimes very acute and painful ones) in the missing limb, confirms the primacy of this sense of body intactness: our deep need to know our bodies not only as whole but as our own. A chief researcher in this field, Ronald Melzack suggests that what we think of as "body image" has a neurological as well as a psychological basis. I find Melzack's hypothesis, that we carry embedded in the very structure of our brains something like a "map" of our bodies, fascinating: it feels so right to me. He postulates that the brain not only receives impulses from the various body parts but generates its own characteristic pattern of impulses "indicating that the body is intact and unequivocally one's own."[6] In other words, despite the fact that the limb is gone, the brain is still wired for wholeness — and I might add, importantly, for symmetry. He also postulates that though this original "map" is unlikely ever to be erased completely, it may be modified over time, as it develops increasingly strong connections with other, still sensate parts of the body which it then begins to serve (p. 124). I find particularly suggestive Melzack's description of how patients who have suffered a lesion of the parietal lobe of the brain, which he postulates as the site the map on which this body-plan is drawn, have pushed a leg outside their hospital bed because they were convinced it belonged to a stranger. The brain map takes precedence, that is, over the evidence of one's own eyes. If a damaged map gives a false reading, tells the body part in question that it is not part of the self, the body will respond to that message rather than to the evidence of its own senses. That account has an eerie resonance with the statements of women so consistently subjected to the top-to-toe inventory of their body parts by others that they have ceased to think of their body parts as belonging to themselves. They are not the victims of amputation; the parts are still there, but they have been "brainwashed" to the point that they no longer know those parts as their own. The map from which the commands are issued is no longer their own.

I have had the opposite, affirmative task to perform, with just one body part, in these last two years — needing to be able to say to the new breast, "this is my body; it is a part of my self." In Melzack's terms, I have had to help the prewired neurosignature accept the new part, the way a body might learn to accept a transplant — even though it was not originally one's own, and even though in this case, it performs none of the physiological functions of the original part. The need to know the new part as one's own, as the phantom limb research suggests, is none the less vital when its function has been exhausted.

Most of the literature, and virtually all of the talk, between doctor and patient engaged in the process of breast reconstruction is centered on how the reconstructed breast will look from the outside. It's on the level of "Will the new lover realize you have a 'reconstructed' breast when you take your clothes off?" But the doctors rarely address the question, "How will it feel?" "Will it feel like part of me?" Everyone else talks about breasts from the outside; I suppose doctors naturally assume that's how women think of their breasts themselves. But they don't — or at least I know now that *I* don't, if I ever did. I remember, sometime when the general sense of having a large wooden box strapped to the left side of my chest began to wear off, tensing my chest muscle, and having the odd sensation that the muscle seemed to have migrated to a new place, above the rounded surface of the new implant, just beneath the skin. It is hard to describe the eeriness of this sensation. I asked my doctor when I next saw him if this were indeed the case, and he casually explained that yes, in order for the implant to be held securely in place, it has to be inserted beneath the chest muscle, which must then itself stretch, along with the skin. What amazed me was his comment that women had never noticed or "complained about" this fact until the present era of "working out" — as if up till then women never knew they had, or had any conscious awareness of having, muscles in their chests at all! Well, maybe. I find it hard to believe women didn't notice. It seems to me more likely that they noticed, but didn't say anything. Perhaps they thought they shouldn't complain; or perhaps they too were primarily thinking about how it looked on the outside and not how it felt on the inside. That, after all, is how we've been taught to think about our bodies, and particularly our most conspicuous sexual parts, our breasts.

What has particularly helped me begin to "recognize" this very different sensation as still my own has been experiencing it through exercise. Exercise, as I indicated earlier, is something I enjoy, something I've used at other critical times in my life as a way of helping me revise my own internal "map" of my body. Moreover, the association between strength and beauty is one I feel helps define me (like many women of my generation) as a feminist. Of course I care about how my breasts look to others and to myself; but I care at least as much about how they feel to me, as parts of my body. I can never recover some of the feelings in the original breast that is no longer there. The sexual feeling, for instance: that's just gone, and I miss it. The new breast might look sexy on the outside, but it doesn't feel sexy on the inside — any more than if I were still of childbearing age it could perform its job of nursing. That knowledge makes me feel sad too. But it doesn't mean that this new breast can't still become part of my body. If I do something I like with those muscles, and if I begin to take care of the new breast (in the shower, for instance, washing it) the way one takes care of any part of one's body, I can begin to make it a real part of my body, a good body, one *I* can love and know as mine.

CHAPTER 7

The Beauty of Age

few months ago, my sister and I, aged fifty-two and fifty-three, were wandering through a crafts fair on Columbus Avenue in New York City. It was the first real spring Sunday afternoon in the city, and New Yorkers were out in all their splendor and diversity, as colorful and tightly packed as the flowers set ouside the Korean groceries. We stopped to look at a bright display of earrings, shiny metal circles with intricate, geometric designs of varied colors and sizes. Trying on one pair after another of these earrings, each with its distinct look (one just right for Judy, we decided in the end, another for me), we became for a happy half-hour or so the curious, interested spectators of our own and each other's appearances. It was, in a way, a reversion to the "dress-up" play of our childhood days in which the pleasure of experimentation and that of self-display each has a part. For many young girls this is a kind of play that extends from childhood on into the fuller discovery of one's sexual self in adolescence; and though for me that line of development was broken, I hope that having recovered it, this is a kind of play I will never lose again — no matter what my age. Indeed I think that, quite aside from the particular insecurities of my own adolescent years, the interest I and many of my contemporary women friends take now in such "dress-up" activity is freer and happier than the equivalent anxiety-laden play (if indeed it can be called "play") of our young womanhood. It's so much easier now to discard the ill-fitting uniform of convention, in this as in other aspects of our lives. I know my own style so much better; and while sisterly advice and affection certainly warmed that particular afternoon's outing for us both, neither Judy or I was thinking of meeting anyone else's expectation of how we ought to look. We left the crafts fair feeling pleased with ourselves and our purchases.

Germaine Greer's brave and in many ways to me inspiring book on the menopause, *The Change: Women, Aging, and the Menopause*,[1] begins with a personal anecdote which also involves a shared experience between the author and an intimate woman friend, each of whom is just turning fifty. There too it is a beautiful spring day, and the two women are enjoying the sensual pleasures of the season — not on Columbus Avenue in New York City but in a café in Beaubourge, France, where, along with their aromatic coffee and buttery croissants, they feast their eyes on the beauty of the flower-filled setting and the fresh season. But the dénouement of Greer's vignette leaves these two fifty-year-old women feeling deeply estranged from rather than in harmony with the glorious spring season blossoming all around them. For abruptly, in the midst of this pleasant interlude in their lives, Greer's friend says to her, "I won't live like that."

> Her eyes were fixed on a little gray lady with a plastic shopping basket apologetically threading her way through the gaudy prostitutes and lounging boys on the pavement opposite. "I won't live in some bedsit with a plate and a knife and a fork and creep out to the market each day for a slice of cheese and a baguette. I won't become gray and invisible. I think what happened to my mother, those years of not knowing where or who she was. I'm not taking that road. I've thought about it. It won't be an unconsidered decision. I don't see the point of the next twenty, thirty years. To get so's your own body makes you sick, no matter how hard you struggle to keep your looks, and keep fit. I can't see the point of battling against it, when you know the outcome can only be defeat. It's so unfair." *(chap. 1, p. 11)*

Greer sees in her friend's panic the irrational "telescoping of the next thirty years into a single grim tomorrow," but admits to having felt a similar sense of panic herself: "Suddenly something was slipping away so fast that we had not had time quite to register what it might be. All we knew was that it was irreplaceable. The way ahead seemed dark." It's life, of course, that's ultimately slipping away here; and that *is* irreplaceable. But the fate we all share as human beings is not what's terrifying these two women at this moment: it's the fate of the old woman in our culture, the "invisible" woman, the "little gray lady," glimpsed across the pavement — the fate of the still living but old woman. And indeed, evidence of the imminence of their own metamorphosis into the person of the "little gray lady" glimpsed across the street is discovered close at hand. At a nearby table two gray-haired men are observed enjoying the adulation of "two sleek expensive, and very much younger women." And so, in their extended fantasy, the two older (obviously more intelligent and more worthy) women see themselves thrust into the unwelcome role of the little gray lady — as invisible to men *of their own age* as Burney's pock-marked Eugenia was to the eligible men of hers: " 'They wouldn't even look at us.' The unkind sunlight showed every sag, every pucker, every bluish shadow, every mole, every freckle in our fifty-year-old faces. When we beckoned to the waiter he seemed not to see us . . ." (p. 12).

I certainly know the outrage Greer and her friend are feeling here, and it is unfair! The disadvantaged status of women in the work world, compounded by the built-in biological disequilibrium between the male and female reproductive systems (not to mention women's greater longevity), all add up to a situation in which women in our society are perceived as sexually superfluous long before men are. And yet, the scenario Greer sketches for us here also makes me uncomfortable. In the first place, how can her companion presume to know what scene of impoverishment or riches that little gray lady may be going home to? And how much sympathy can I feel for women who lament the fact that they are invisible to total strangers — and, on the evidence, rather unappealing ones? Isn't the anxiety of these two upper-class, fifty-year-old women really about the loss of a special kind of elitist status? Wouldn't one rather step around a prostitute than be one?

Elsewhere in her book Greer's references to a young woman's

sexuality are curiously anonymous. She never draws a persuasive portrait of a young woman whose sexuality is linked to feelings of self-discovery and self-love. You are left to wonder whether what she and her companion are being forced to give up in this initial vignette has everything to do with power and nothing to do with love. The post-menopausal woman, as Greer presents her, is a woman whom men "no longer sniff around," whom they no longer "bother to intimidate . . . by whistles and catcalls as she passes the building site" (p. 52). And she may, understandably enough, discover she misses a kind of attention she didn't like when she had it: "She had not realized how much she depended upon her physical presence, at shop counters, at the garage, on the bus." Perhaps because I *didn't* (and couldn't) depend on that sort of attention as a young woman, I can only see that sort of visibility as something not worth the candle. The problem for me is that Greer seems to equate this sort of superficial and elitist visibility with sexuality, or a life in the body, itself. And thus in urging women to let go of it, she asks us to give up too much.

Greer's alternate scenario to the one pictured in this opening scene — the life she portrays in her book as a whole and invites the post-menopausal woman not simply to accept but embrace — insofar as it is a life rich in mental reflection and outward-turning actions, is one that requires no special pleading as far as I'm concerned. It's a wonderful life! I too would rather embrace the opportunities of age than make an (ultimately doomed) effort to hold onto the pleasures of youth. And it's true that the post-childbearing years do offer (some) women in our society an opportunity to lead a freer life in the spirit. But do we really want to see these years as a time when a woman can "change back into the self [she was] before [she] became a tool of [her] sexual and reproductive destiny" (p. 55)?[2] This sounds more like a retreat than an advance to me. Does the extension of a woman's spiritual life in age have to be predicated on a corresponding shrinkage of her previous life in the body? Aren't women's needs, in *both* stages of their lives, shortchanged by such an antithesis? At one point Greer herself suggests that what the post-menopausal woman is really afraid of losing with "the change" is not her status as a sex object, which (willingly or not) she must forgo, but something more precious, and something she cannot lose: her essential female identity, difficult as that may be to define (p. 52). I only wish we could hear more here about how that essential femaleness which, as she says, "the onset and retreat of a woman's reproductive years cannot alter," colors in all sorts of intangible yet meaningful ways the life of the post- as well as a pre-menopausal woman.

If we are ready now, as I believe many women in my generation are, to see beauty and sexual identity in the old woman as well as the young one, where can we find the role models who will help us to see this shadowy figure more clearly, and show us how in our turn we might become her? When I ask my middle-aged women friends how they feel about the aging of their own bodies, they generally respond — just as Greer's friend in the café does — with some allusion to their own mothers' aging. And of course the prospect of our own aging scares us, when, for most of us, as for Greer's friend, what we saw was anything but affirming! Not that our mothers said much (if anything) to us about their experiences of aging, other than a muttered complaint about an aching back or "the size 10 dress I used to wear." Not one of my contemporaries recalls her mother speaking to her in personal terms about the experience of menopause. But, particularly for those of us with older mothers, we whose mothers' reproductive years were close to ending just as our own were starting, the unspoken message about women's aging came through loud and clear.

In my own case, the negative message came, not from a mother whose life had largely been defined, like those of the mothers of most of my friends, by issues of "marriage and family . . . body and beauty" (in Betty Friedan's terms),[3] but from one deeply committed to her professional life. The beauty question isn't, as it is too often assumed to be, only an issue for women who have nothing else "going for them" in their lives. I remember as an adolescent watching my stepmother, then in her late forties, applying lipstick with what appeared to be deliberate carelessness (the lipstick never came out even, really not even close), and then, with an expression somewhere between a shrug and a grimace, glance at her reflection in the mirror. "I may have been an attractive woman once," that glance seemed to say, "but not any more." I didn't understand why she should be so dismissive of her appearance. To be sure, I hadn't known her as a young woman (she was forty-two when she entered my life as my father's new wife and our new mother). And I could see that she must have been a very beautiful young girl: an elegant not-quite-profile photograph taken when she was in her mid-teens, mounted on the wall along the stairway, showed finely cut features, dark, fashionably cropped hair, and an earnest and yet hopeful look — which somehow reminded me of the picture on the cover of one of my favorite books, *The Diary of Anne Frank*. But to me my stepmother was also an attractive woman now — the more so, no doubt, because her beauty was of a style I could never hope to achieve. When I looked at the face I knew, I saw a small-boned "classical" beauty of feature and large, intelligent, if often sad-seeming eyes. The signs of aging which were evidently so conspicuous to her didn't register with me at all. And I was distressed as well as puzzled by that self-deprecating gesture. I must have longed for her to show me that she still did care for her appearance, partly to help me learn how to care for my own newly female body. But for reasons I didn't understand, she wouldn't do it.

Now that I am myself the age she was then, I think I understand better the reasons behind her refusal. But if I do understand better, that's not because I too now know how it feels to have sagging skin and graying hair. It's rather because I'm more conscious of the extent to which one's response to the aging of one's body is intertwined with everything else that is going on in one's life at the same time. Playing back that lipstick scene now, I realize that the dismissive gesture I saw was really an expression of anger at and, beneath that, some underlying disappointment in my father. He probably would not have noticed and certainly would not have been bothered by a wife who wore no lipstick. But he was very much bothered by a wife who put on make-up (and articles of dress generally) with an evident carelessness. And my father was particularly proud of his own strikingly youthful appearance: at forty-eight he had virtually no grey hair, while hers was almost entirely grey. In some relationships it might not have mattered, or might not have placed him at an advantage; it is perfectly possible for grey, or white, hair to seem very beautiful. But in their relationship it did matter. Well, if he were going to make so much of his youthful appearance, she would retaliate by making, as it were, the most of her age.

The lipstick vignette tempts me to generalize that a seeming indifference to or disdain for one's body is, just as much in age as in youth, a distress signal. *If* it were possible for us to believe there is nothing intrinsically unattractive about an older body, then we might be more attuned to such distress signals, less willing to write them off with some glib phrase, such as, "Well, naturally she's just feeling disappointed about losing her looks." (As if a look could be lost!) Or worse, "Good for her; she knows better than to fuss over her appearance. She's put all that nonsense behind her." Perhaps, *if* we could see the aging body through a different lens, then a woman who finds herself chronicling (in adolescent fashion) every defect of her aging body might explore further the real source of her distress, which is likely to be more than skin-deep. Consider, for example, the distress evident in this speech from Doris Grumbach's "Coming into the End Zone": "Now I look, hard. I see the pull of gravity on the soft tissues of my breasts and buttocks. I see the heavy rings that encircle my neck like Ubangi jewelry. I notice bones that seem to have thinned and shrunk. Muscles appear to be watered down. The walls of my abdomen, like Jericho, have softened and now press outward. There is nothing lovely about the sight of me."[4] It's natural to respond in sympathy to the distress in this voice, isn't it, by suggesting there is another way to understand — to see — the aging female body?

Grumbach goes on to say in the wonderfully honest piece from which I have just quoted, "I have been taught that firm and unlined is beautiful. Shall I try to learn to love what I am left with? I wonder.

It would be easier to resolve never again to look into a full-length mirror." She's right; it is what we've all been taught — and are still being taught. Advertisers for skin creams pander to our fantasy that aging skin is nothing more than a mistake, and one that can be corrected:

> When skin persists in showing lines, signs of past sun damage, poor texture, muddiness, dullness, Clinique pronounces it perfect.
>
> Perfect because this kind of skin is the ideal candidate for a remarkable new skin corrector, Clinique Turnaround Cream.
>
> Fact is [!] your skin has a younger version of itself deep inside and Turnaround Cream's job is to help this fresh layer surface — renewed, de-aged, de-flaked, old mistakes left behind come morning.   (New Yorker, *August 16, 1993*)

The "real" me (the youthful me) is just waiting there to be excavated! This would be merely funny — but that one knows such an advertisement and others like it wouldn't exist if they didn't sell the product, and didn't therefore give voice to the self-contempt of the aging woman in our culture.

At my twenty-fifth college reunion some years ago there seemed to be a general consensus among the assembled women then in their late forties that on the whole we looked *better* than we had twenty-five years ago. The signs of aging that as individuals in our private lives we generally read so negatively (grey hair, wrinkle marks) were certainly evident; but on this occasion we were not perceiving them in one another as repellent or distressing. What this experience tells me is not that the survivors of the Bryn Mawr College class of 1962 are a particularly hardy or "well-preserved" group of women. It tells me that in this particular *context* we could perceive the signs of aging in positive rather than negative terms. And what was that context? A reunion of women who had in common their attendance at a woman's college known then as now for taking women students seriously (never mind the abysmal career counseling in those days!); and, in the present setting, the virtual absence of men. I suspect that such a perception of aging women's bodies as attractive would have been, at the least, much harder to come by, had we been graduates returning to a co-educational institution. We were, perhaps, in this context, enabled to see our beauty in the same way that a new audience of educated women readers in the late eighteenth and nineteenth centuries was enabled by some great, imaginative women writers to see their own beauty in new terms.

My nineteenth-century fictions, however — limited as they are to a definition of the heroine as a young, marriageable woman — cannot help me in my search for an image of women who are perceived as beautiful in either middle-age or genuine old age. In the fiction of our own century I can, however, think of several compelling older-women-heroines whom we see struggling with if not necessarily resolving the issues of women's aging. There is Kate Brown in Doris Lessing's 1973 novel, *The Summer Before the Dark* (a novel interestingly discussed by Greer).[5] And there is a wonderful description of the not exactly old but aging body of Frances Wingate, the heroine of Drabble's 1975 novel, *The Realms of Gold*, as we see it "reduced," for purposes of memory, "into a series of images," by her absent lover — a description I can't resist quoting here, in part because it suggests that novelists often grow up (as Drabble does) along with their heroes or heroines. Here is Sarah of *A Summer Bird-Cage*, her skin no longer firm and unblemished, but with flesh to be celebrated all the more because it shows the marks of time, and, more specifically, of the particular life she has lived. The thirty-some-year-old Frances Wingate is an anthropologist, and her lover's description of her body appropriately shares in the anthropologist's delight in discovering the marks wrought by time:

> First of all, he would think of the color of her. She was brown and
> yellow. Her skin was golden, and it was an interesting mixture of
> coarseness and sensitivity: it had been weathered, as she was fond
> of pointing out, by sun and sand, like an ancient monument. She
> was covered in blemishes: scars, rough patches, corns, permanently

damaged nails, moles, and a large brown birthmark on her bottom. He would think of these details, one after the other. Then he would think of making love to her and how much she seemed to like it.[6]

It is in a film, however, rather than a work of fiction, that I find my best model for the beautiful yet truly old woman. And I have chosen a film in this instance in part because I want a model here that does more than give us an image of beauty we can hold in our mind's eye—something more than such words, wonderful as they are, with which Shakespeare "fleshes out" his affirmation that Cleopatra's beauty is such that "age cannot wither . . . nor custom stale / Her infinite variety." On the stage Shakespeare's Cleopatra was a young boy; the physical image couldn't carry it—which is partly why the language, which does carry it, is all the more persuasive. But in this instance, just because the resistance in our culture to the possibility of seeing beauty in the old woman is so strong, I want the physical image itself—shaped to be sure by the filmmaker's own vision, yet an image we can actually see with our eyes. A great actress playing the part of Jane Eyre in a film version of that novel would take her cue from Brontë's text and find ways to help us gradually see Jane becoming beautiful, as she gains Rochester's love and as we get to know her and love her better ourselves. But I think it is fair to say that, while it would be a pleasure to see such a performance, Jane Eyre *needs* that sort of attention less. After all, however "plain" Jane may be, the very fact of her youth automatically defines her as marriageable and therefore, seen through those lenses of conventions we scarcely know we wear but find almost impossible to take off, potentially beautiful. A woman past the age of fifty is not eligible in that sense. If we're really going to teach ourselves to see the beauty in an old woman, then I think it helps actually to *see* them, so we feel we know the truth of their beauty first hand. This means that I'm not only asking you to read what I have to say about this film; I'm also asking you to see it (it's available on video), and to see it again if you've already seen it once.

The film is *Strangers in Good Company*, a Canadian film released in 1990 (1991 in the U.S.). Using all nonprofessional actresses, it gained a large (and to its makers unexpected) public following as well as critical acclaim — though the New York reviewers were content to pronounce it merely "charming." In fact the reception of this film, as well as the actresses' (or participants') responses to that reception, seems to mimic traditional responses to and of old women themselves. "Modest and appealing," says Janet Maslin (*New York Times*, May 10, 1991). "It sneaks up on you like your first gray hair," says Rita Kempley (*Washington Post*, July 13, 1991); and from the women in the film the amazed response to its huge success, *their* success: "Is it possible? Can they really like us?"

The film is a "semi-documentary" about the lives of seven women, the youngest of whom is sixty-five and the oldest of whom is eighty-eight. One young woman, aged twenty-seven, is also present — but she's a foil for the older women and does not occupy the space on this set that the young woman generally preempts for herself: center stage. In fact, this young woman is interestingly incapacitated near the start of the film and becomes therefore the one figure in the film whose movements are severely restricted. This is going to be a film about *old* women.

The original screenplay for *Strangers in Good Company* (or *The Company of Strangers* in its original Canadian title) called for a group of elderly women tourists, en route to "a Golden Age exchange program," whose bus breaks down somewhere in the Canadian wilderness (the one young woman is the driver of the bus). The women spend three days in and around an abandoned farmhouse, while they devise various rescue schemes, work at survival, and (most importantly) get to know one another. Finally, the youngest of the old women (Catherine) goes out to scout for help, succeeds in reaching civilization, and returns in a helicopter to rescue the others. But this is not an action film; despite the catastrophic possibilities inherent in the situation, there's virtually no dramatic suspense, and the effect of being suspended in a timeless world is enhanced by the fact that we're given very little detail about such practical matters as what happens when. In fact in the final version of the film we are not told where these women were originally headed in their bus, how well (if at all) they may have known one another at the start, or exactly how long a time period passes before their rescue.

One can't but contemplate how different a film involving men of the same age group would have to be if it were to have any credibility! But to this group of women what matters is not the final rescue or any of the actions that might lead up to it. In a book on the making of the film, Mary Meigs, herself a member of the cast, describes the world of the film in these terms:

> the mist from which we emerge at the beginning of the film . . .
> symbolizes the absence of explanation. The audience is asked to be-
> lieve that none is needed; the mist cuts us off from reasons, and lifts
> to show us, who have stepped out of time and logic into *a magic
> space where old women have room to exist.* We are, at the time of film-
> ing: Alice Diabo, 74; Constance Garneau, 88; Winifred Holden, 76;
> Cissy Meddings, 76; Mary Meigs, 71; Catherine Roche, 65; Beth
> Webber, 80.[7]

"A magic space where old women have room to exist." That says it perfectly, reminding us that no such place exists in the real world. Meigs's book is a meditation on the film and its meaning for all the women involved in it — some of whom had responded to an advertisement in a Montreal newspaper, others of whom had been specifically solicited by the directors. The passage I've just quoted, taken as a whole, suggests that if the space the film occupies is a magic space, the women in it are not magical at all: they are very real women, with real names and ages. What's magical is the gift of being allowed, through the medium of the film and filmmakers' love, to see these women as they truly are.

Although the original screenplay for *Strangers* by Gloria Demers contained a certain amount of dialogue, the film as originally conceived by Demers and Cynthia Scott called for the women, once established in their fictive world, to play themselves and to enact their own drama. The directors had faith that, in the process, what emerged would in some manner or other constitute a tribute to women's lives. The film does so — without any propagandizing, but simply by revealing. We see the women cutting the tall grass to make mattresses to sleep on, catching fish in an improvised pantyhose net, trying to fix the bus, sending up smoke-signals. These activities have the function which, in a normal gathering of women, sewing might, or watching the children play in the park: they are essential, or required, activities. But their more important function is to provide a stage on which the real action can take place: the conversation. The women talk — for the most part in small groups of two or three — about their lives and the people with whom they've shared their lives. At several points they touch upon their fears of death and abandonment. And in one scene several of them speculate as to whether they could fall in love again: "You're still alive. . . . You don't lose interest just because you're getting older." *You're still alive.* That's a refrain that echoes through the film. "Is anybody there? We're alive!" at one point the women, standing together, call out to the surrounding mountains, and again, "We're alive!" Their cry is as much an affirmation of what they are, here on their own, as it is a plea for help.

One of the most moving scenes in the film is an unscripted conversation between Michelle (the young bus driver) and Beth, at eighty one of the oldest members of the group. As Meigs points out, Michelle personifies the vibrancy and energy of youth in the film — even with the "sprained ankle" which, in the plot's fiction, prevents her from playing a caretaking role in relation to the old women — or, more accurately, allows *their* energy, with its very different rhythms, to come through. Impulsive, curious, sympathetic, loud (a jazz singer in real life), Michelle wears her cloud of black hair pulled back from her face with a pink scarf. Beth, on the other hand, stands out among the old women as the most carefully put together (or covered up) of the group, the only one who seems uncomfortable, even in this setting, with the fact of her age. We see her, on waking from her bed of straw, reach anxiously for her purse, touch her hair to assure herself that all is as it should be, then taking her compact from the purse, study her face in its mirror.

The scene between these two women, one old and one young,

is about self-exposure — particularly but not merely the exposure of the body. Or maybe it would be more accurate to say that when we expose our bodies there is a strong feeling that we are exposing our whole self with it. If we think back to Freud's notion of sco-pophilia, the natural pleasure taken (particularly though not exclusively) by a man in seeing the sexual parts of a member of the opposite sex, and the complementary pleasure she (or perhaps he) takes in having those parts seen, we might add that in a social context both these pleasures may be charged with some degree of anxiety. He may be wondering whether his overture will be rejected, or whether he may be distressed (frightened?) by what he sees. And she may be feeling even more vulnerable. She wants to reveal herself to the man; but what if she does so, and her gift of herself is rejected?

An old woman who covers up her body to the extent that Beth does in this film is not showing indifference to her appearance or to how others may respond to it — particularly if she is (like Beth) a woman who enjoyed frequent compliments on her appearance when she was younger. She is expressing her fear that if she exposes herself she may be courting a painful rejection. There is a special tenderness, then, as the drama of exposure and loving acceptance is played out here, not between a man and a woman, but between two women. The old woman feels a safety she would not feel with a man in exposing her body *as it is* to this friendly young woman: Michelle will be in Beth's place, an old woman too in her turn, and both women know that.

The scene begins with Beth telling Michelle she envies her vivacity and the energy she perceives in the other women despite their age, and Michelle urges her to "loosen up," "let yourself go." Beth responds by laughing and saying that it's a little late for her to begin trying out a whole new style of life. Michelle comments that she could at least take off her shoes (high heels) or unbutton her shirt a bit. Beth, fingering the top button of her tailored shirt, says with a new frankness, "Well, shall I tell you why I keep this buttoned? I don't want my wrinkled neck to show." They both laugh at the foolishness of feminine vanity — but the shirt remains buttoned.

Then, turning the encounter into a parody of male-female strip-tease, but also one in which the two women share in the act of disclosure, Michelle takes her own scarf off her head and, running her hand through her springing hair, extends an invitation to Beth, "Come on. You take something off. I'll take something off." The warmth in Michelle's smile lets us know she is on Beth's side, sure that there could be nothing about Beth's aging body that would better be hidden. "Well, I took my *jacket* off" Beth says, "I thought I was being . . ." her voice fading out. Michelle, now emboldened, points toward Beth's hair, and declares, "This has got to go." And if we hadn't realized it before, we see now that Beth's neat little cap of gray-brown hair is a wig. Beth demurs: she says she's tried, but she can't go without "the damn thing." Michelle offers to tie Beth's hair up in her own pink scarf, but to her repeated invitations, Beth replies, "Oh . . . I don't know. I don't think so." And then, testing: "I may surprise you any minute though." "Shock me," Michelle invites her. "Would it be a shock?" Beth asks, with gaining confidence. "O.K., I'll shock you." And with a gesture at once tentative and impulsive (like a child leaping into the water she fears may drown her), Beth abruptly pulls off her wig.

For an instant she looks inquiringly, with something very close to terror, at Michelle, uncertain of the latter's response. And for that instant the viewer (or this viewer) feels a kindred horror, as the mask of youth is stripped away and the head of the old crone is exposed, her pathetically thin wisps of colorless hair accentuating the contour of the skull and the large, frightened eyes. But the instant is no more than that. For as Beth sees Michelle's warm smile and hears her "It looks beautiful!" relief floods her face. She smiles in her turn, and suddenly we see what Michelle has seen, a beautiful woman delighting in the revelation of herself. Next, Michelle hands her scarf to Beth who, maidenlike, hesitates — "I haven't got any hair. I did enough. Don't get mad with me"; but then, with the sure touch of an expert, she winds the scarf about her head, leaving a bit of her white hair visible at the crown, brings the ends forward around her neck, and with a little flourish of her hand, flips one end of the scarf over her shoulder. Patting the sides of her head, affectionately now, she smiles the smile of a proud woman, who is at the same time making fun of her vanity. The two women laugh. "Fantastic!" says Michelle with a broad grin, and it is.

Beth's disclosure of her unwigged self leads her to a parallel disclosure in conversation with Michelle. She shares her experience of growing up in a poor family, admits her regrets at never having had a formal education (which makes her feel inferior), and also reveals the source of her life's greatest happiness, and tragedy — her son, who died at the age of twenty-seven. "I've never been happy since then," she admits. Michelle asks more questions about this loved child; there is a pause. "I don't even want to talk about it," says Beth, "it's . . . it's still too painful." And the scene draws to a close.

In its closing, the scene offers a recognition of the need for boundaries. We might have thought we'd seen the last of Beth's wig, but when she appears in later scenes the wig is back in place. Her wearing it is a reminder that this *is* a special place where in special moments the unguardedness of intimacy is possible, but that these women — both in their real and in their fictive lives — will soon be returning to the world.

From Meigs's book we learn that the drama of Beth's temporary removal of her wig was reenacted on the set, off-camera. On the evening of the day on which the scene between Beth and Michelle was filmed Beth appeared at the dinner table of the resort hotel at which the cast and filmmakers were staying: "'Beth, you look wonderful!' everybody says. Without her wig she has a very high forehead and her eyes seem huge, bright and haunted. The next day Beth is wearing her wig again" (pp. 52–53). Even in the semi-sheltered world of the set, and the more sheltered one of the film, the real world is never entirely forgotten. Beth is not going to gain enough confidence, we realize, from these moments, to bring back all of her real self into the world.

Cynthia Scott had hoped to include a scene of larger self-

exposure in the film: the women were to have gone swimming naked in the lake. And that too might have been a wonderfully liberating scene — to break through the taboo against revealing old
women's bodies, and help us see that they, in their very wornness,
can be beautiful. "But weather didn't permit and the lake got too
cold" Meigs tells us (p. 74). So instead what we see are the women,
fully clothed, splashing one another, like children, in the stream.
Could these wonderfully loving and encouraging directors have
pulled off a nude scene? I'm not sure — the members of the cast
themselves were very resistant to the idea, and their tension (if it
hadn't dissipated) would have spoiled it. But I agree with Meigs
when she acknowledges, speaking perhaps as an artist rather than a
subject, that, for all her personal relief that it didn't come off,
"[Cynthia] knows and I know that it would have been a beautiful
scene" (p. 74). And I'm sorry it's not there.

In *Strangers* the natural wilderness setting is used to frame and
help define the women's beauty. Seen in this world where growth
and decay each has its place, the old women's wrinkled skin can't
register, like that in the magazine ads, as "mistakes." Especially in
the scenes featuring Constance, the oldest of the women, one feels
an intimate relation between the human figure and the landscape.
Constance, a woman of great reserve and dignity, stands always
somewhat apart from the group, looking out at the landscape, and
she is the one who ventures forth into it — not in search of rescue
from outside, but in search of something *in* this special world.
(Even though we don't know the women's destination when the
film opens, we do know the bus made the detour from the main
road onto the smaller one, on which it broke down, in order to grat-
ify Constance's wish to see once more her childhood summer
home. At some point after that first night, we see her, cane in hand,
laboriously descending the farmhouse porch stairs. Slowly, pur-
posefully, she makes her way through the field, as the camera pans
back to show her form partly obscured by the tall grasses, the soft
white of her hair and dress at home in the vast field's pale yellow.
And as she crosses (still moving very slowly) a small stone bridge

by the border of the nearby lake, the camera shows not the woman
herself but her diffused image as it is reflected in the water, enhanc-
ing the effect of a merger between the human figure and the landscape. Eventually, we see her pause and look intently at a small
house on the far shore. Then at last she stands, at rest, at its porch
railing, looking out over the water. The camera lingers, first on
her figure in the landscape, then, in slow panorama, on the expanse
of lake, mountains, and sky, as she sees it, looking outward, and
finally rests on her face, quiet, intently watching. We realize that
Constance has found her childhood home, the place of her former
happiness. But we also realize, as she looks out over the still water
—and then again later, when she very deliberately spills all her
pills into the water—that she has found the place in which to die.
"It makes me happy," she says of the setting later, "even if it's
only for a little while." And again, "I'm going to die pretty soon
anyway. Rather die here than in a nursing home." That human
death can be acknowledged in this world and placed in the context
of nature's life, is one of the things that make it possible for us to
see the beauty in these old women. For our sense of the ugliness
of the old is, at bottom, a fear of death. And in nature, where it is
part of the cycle of birth and decay, the individual death, loses its
terror.

Nature is everywhere in this film, and men are absent. (Here the
ban is absolute: even when Catherine leans out from the rescuing
helicopter, shouting, "I made it! I made it!" the features of the helicopter's pilot are obscured from our view.) It is worth pondering
further why this ban seems necessary, why when in all my other
models for a beauty that's hard to perceive, it is still the beloved man
who draws it out and validates it for the woman. Why should it be
otherwise here? I think for the simple reason that the question of
women's beauty is not, even implicitly, linked here to the issue of
procreation, and thus to all those assumptions about the ownership
of women's bodies by men which color our feelings about beauty
(and even about sexual desirability) in our daily lives in the world.
This is not to say that a man *watching* the film would be less likely
to respond positively to the beauty of these women: in fact, it was

the man with whom I first saw this film who pointed out to me the beauty of these women and speculated about its source. But were a man to be present *in* the film, his very presence would create the atmosphere of appraisal which would make it at best difficult for the viewer (and perhaps for the members of the cast themselves) to see these women for what they are and to celebrate their beauty.

In this context it is certainly important that the film celebrates the lesbian woman as well as the elderly one. In her book Meigs suggests that for each of the women there was a particular scene "that required an act of courage, one that would only be possible in that atmosphere of trust" (p. 52), and the disclosure of her own lesbianism is that scene for her. In fact, as she explains in the book, the directors had selected her in part because they wanted the film to make a statement about lesbianism. Celebrating lesbianism and celebrating old women go together: they are the two most conspicuous groups of women in our society cut loose from the patriarchal structure (especially as old women are so much more likely to be living independently than men). Seeing the film, we understand why the directors wanted Mary to be what she calls wryly the film's "token lesbian": hers is such a strong, articulate, and affirmative presence. It is, to begin with, the physical presence which draws our attention from the very start of the film. Mary is the outstanding "picture-book" beauty of the group, with elegant, finely cut features, penetrating eyes, and a warm (often wry, self-mocking) smile. Her full head of white hair and the lines at the corners of her eyes and mouth are aspects of her beauty — impossible for anyone to read these as "mistakes." Moreover it is Mary who tends to assume something like a narrator's role in the film's action, just as in its real-life aftermath she is the one who assumed responsibility for the continuing life of the group as a whole, becoming both its chronicler and interpreter to the world at large.

The directors knew they wanted some sort of lesbian "statement" in the film, but they didn't know how or when it should take place; nor did Mary herself — who was not, she tells us, altogether comfortable with the role of lesbian representative on the set. What makes it work, though, is the naturalness of the "statement" when it "just happens," beautifully, in a scene between Mary and Cissy. Lovable, persistently cheerful, and deep-down indomitable, with a small, round not-so-finely-strung body, a lilting, high-pitched voice, and colorful, emphatically cockney speech, Cissy is Mary's physical and social opposite.

The two women are birdwatching together in the large, open field. Mary has referred to the fact that it's the male bird who generally does the singing—females rarely sing—though occasionally a pair will sing together, in duet. "Oh lovely!" Cissy exclaims in her high-pitched voice, listening. They return to their birdwatching, and then Cissy (following the natural path of her associations) looks at Mary again, pauses, and asks, "Do you live alone, Mary?" "No. Well, I do at the moment, yes. But I've spent a lot of my life living with other women." And Cissy, puzzled, says, "Do you? Not a man friend?" "Never a man, no." Still not getting it, Cissy asks "Oh, why not?" The inquiry is so warm, so innocent, Mary can't help smiling as she responds, "Oh, you know, Cissy, I'm a lesbian. I don't really like . . . men don't interest me. I've had my little experiments, but (wryly), they didn't work out. I get along better with women." And Cissy, echoing, accepting, "Women . . . Oh, that's good." And the camera follows the path of a bird across the field as the two women turn back to their birdwatching. (Here's an instance in which a human life-pattern departs from nature's.)

When we come back to them, we see that the two women are no longer standing but are seated next to one another on the crates they have brought out for that purpose. Cissy, curious, returns to the subject: "Did it alter your life in any way, your turning from one to the other?" Mary explains that she didn't "turn": she was what she was all along. It was very hard, though, in her generation—the "secret generation." But when Cissy responds with the naive affirmation, "*You* weren't ashamed, were you?" Mary says that indeed she *was* ashamed. "You had to be. Everybody disapproved." Cissy understands better now and makes her own contribution: "You hid behind the closet door," at which the two women laugh together conspiratorially. Mary continues, explaining that once she had broken her silence — which only happened after she was sixty — she began writing about her lesbianism, and now, she confesses, she can't stop. "Good idea," says Cissy. "Why should you stop?" "Why should I? Everybody's life is more or less interesting." "It's a drama," Cissy agrees. And at that point the conversation shifts to the drama of her own life, specifically to her willed recovery from a severe stroke.

One wonders whether Mary's earlier secretiveness about her lesbianism was not a function of her age as well as of the style of her generation. For in this film we're struck again and again how these women, freed from both the intense involvements and obligations of earlier years, feel they can — in this company — declare themselves, in ways both large and small. Catherine can say in this secular company that she is a nun, and explain why. Cissy and Alice can share their feelings of being abandoned in their old age. Beth can confess her embarrassment about her wrinkled neck and her continuing grief for the loss of her son. Constance can weep, realizing the imminence of her own death. And Alice and Winnie can recall together the intense sexual pleasures of their youth and admit that they might still be able to feel such things again: " . . . if the right guy came along." "Why not?" "I suppose." "We've still got our hopes and dreams." These old women are, as they tell us in so many ways, in their distinctive voices, alive — and perhaps *more* so than they were in earlier days, because they are more fully themselves and more accepting of themselves, and this is the source of their beauty.

Meigs plays with the correspondences and the differences between the "company of strangers" *making* the film and the "company of strangers" *in* the film:

> In reality, we are seven old women and a young woman. People look curiously at us as we file into the Riviere Rouge for lunch, or they stare openly at us, for we look to them just like seven old women, some of us not entirely steady on our feet. And what are we doing there? One day, after three oafish, unshaven men in checked shirts and muddy boots have been too engrossed in staring

even to drink their beer, Winnie says wryly, "I wanted to say to them, 'What are you staring at? Haven't you ever seen film stars before?'" The three men didn't know that we were film stars disguised as old women. *(p. 34)*

The truth, however, is more complex. They *are* "film stars," in the sense that it is only through the lens of art that we can perceive their beauty; and they are "old women" who, by definition, are objects of ridicule to "oafish" men.

Meigs comments on the shock the cast members felt when they first viewed the film. Their experience was in a sense the opposite of that of the viewers: for what they saw was the revelation of themselves as old women. She observes: "We stick with an interior image, the young woman sitting at the edge of the pool, even when her hair turns grey, then white . . . 'Do I look like that? You've made me look so old.' . . . 'So that's the way I look!' 'That dreary old woman.'" Most of us in our age call up the real or imagined snapshots of youth; so it is not surprising that for Meigs seeing again in the finished film the photographs that intermittently flash across the screen and interrupt the present narrative to show us each woman as she was in earlier days is a wrenching experience: "I ache with the pain of seeing what we were long ago, when every one of us was beautiful with the beauty of a child or a young person full of careless energy" (p. 76).

But for me as a spectator of the film, the effect of those childhood and young-womanhood photographs — though equally powerful — is exactly the reverse of what it is for Mary Meigs as a participant. I, who know these women only as old women, and who have seen the expressiveness in their bodies in motion, see those still, childhood photos as less real, less persuasive. Some of them are indeed lovely images in themselves: little Beth, with the classic heart-shaped face and bow lips; Catherine, as a novice, smiling, with a mane of long golden hair; Mary herself, innocent and intense; Cissy, in the embrace of her devoted husband (now dead). A reviewer of the film assumes that these early photos are there to prove to us that these old women were beautiful — once. And perhaps that was the intention of the directors. But for me they constitute the most powerful possible validation of the filmmakers' art, which, overturning one of our culture's most powerful conventions, has made the old woman more beautiful than the young one.

That such moments of vision as these should be possible is, to me, exilarating. To know that we can get this far away from those images of beauty instilled in us by the culture in which we all live is profoundly affirming. For if we can see the beauty in the old face as well as the young one, in the black face as well as the white one, see the beauty in any face that speaks to us of love or is informed by our own love, then we are taking off old blinders. We are seeing the world and its beauty, as Jane Eyre describes the way Rochester's love allows him to see her, with "eyes new-dyed." Such seeing, subjectively based as it is, is also the truest seeing. In the imaginative worlds of *Strangers in Good Company* and Drabble's *Realms of Gold*, of Morrison's *The Bluest Eye*, and in the diverse nineteenth-century women's fictions I have been discussing in these pages, it is the artist's eye that enables us to see the world thus new-dyed. But through the aid of such imaginative lenses we can then begin to see human beauty anew in the world in which we actually live from day to day — in our own faces and, equally importantly, in all the varied faces of others.

In *Strangers in Good Company* the discovery of beauty in the old woman's body is possible only in a world that is twice removed from reality — first, by the artificiality imposed by the film form, and second, by the removal of the characters from the world of society to that of a nature that is in harmony with the life-rhythms of their bodies. And the nineteenth-century fictions in which I have sought and found my own best models for the reclamation of the beauty of my own person are also, of course, removed from reality — again by the distancing of art, and further, by that of time. It seems to me, however, that, as feminists, using one another's experience as our models, we should be ready now to entertain the possibility of such seeing in the real world — both, that is, in our own varied, psychic worlds and in the larger social world we all inhabit.

The reclamation of personal beauty I am proposing in this book is an invitation to join in a liberating venture. It is not antithetical to a woman's (or a man's) pursuit of what Heilbrun calls a "quest" life — a life that takes its meaning from some action pursued in the public world. But it asks us to recover — or better, to reinvent — an area of experience which, as feminists, many of us have felt we needed to abandon. It asks us to see with eyes new-dyed the beauty of our own bodies. And that means, whatever our race or age or outward aspect, that we have the strength to claim ownership of our own bodies. But it also means that we have the strength to honor and celebrate the passive experience of being there for another person, to recognize the beauty of "presence." Both aspects of this more private quest seem to me ventures that we, as feminists, are ready now to undertake.

Notes

Chapter 1. *The Beauty Myths*

1.   Toni Morrison, *The Bluest Eye* (New York: Simon & Schuster, Pocket Books, 1970), p. 34.

2.   Baldesar Castiglione, *The Book of the Courtier*, trans. Charles S. Singleton (Garden City, N.Y.: Doubleday & Company, Inc., Anchor Books, 1959), pp. 342–43.

3.   I have taken the term "beauty myth" from Naomi Wolf's recent book, *The Beauty Myth: How Images of Beauty are Used Against Women* (New York: Morrow & Company, Inc., 1991). Wolf's version of the beauty myth is discussed later in this chapter and, more fully, in chapter 2.

4.   Susan Brownmiller, *Femininity* (1984; New York: Fawcett Columbine, Ballantine Books, 1985), pp. 40–41.

5.   See the discussion of the nineteenth-century feminist "purity crusade" and the legacy of ambivalence about sexual liberation it created for a later generation of feminists in Judith R. Walkowitz, "Male Vice and Female Virtue: Feminism and the Politics of Prostitution in Nineteenth-Century Britain," in *Desire: The Politics of Sexuality*, ed. Ann Snitow, Christine Stansell, and Sharon Thompson (London: Virago Press Limited, 1983), pp. 43–61.

6.   *A Vindication of the Rights of Women* (1792), vol. 5 in *The Works of Mary Wollstonecraft*, ed. Janet Todd and Marilyn Butler (assistant ed. Emma Rees-Mogg), 7 vols (London: William Pickering & Chatto, 1958), p. 113.

7.   Brownmiller, *Femininity*, pp. 50–51.

8.   This assumption that women live within a world in which the "shared" language is not their language (or cannot express what they would wish to say) is particularly associated with French feminism; but the question of language, and the possibilities of women's speech within a patriarchal society are major concerns of American feminist critics as well. For a good review of this issue see Mary Jacobus's introductory essay ("The Difference in View," pp. 10–21)

and the essays collected in the anthology, *Women Writing and Writing About Women*, ed. Jacobus (New York: Barnes & Noble, 1979). For the problem of women's speech about their own bodies see particularly Helena Michie, *The Flesh Made Word: Female Figures and Women's Bodies* (New York and Oxford: Oxford University Press, 1987). This is a stimulating study, from which I have learned much. But I am more optimistic than Michie and some other contemporary feminists about the capacity of language (any language) to express feeling. The corollary notion that women must, in effect, invent a whole new language to express their feelings informs the collection of essays assembled in *The Female Body in Western Culture: Contemporary Perspectives*, ed. Susan Rubin Suleiman (Cambridge, Mass.: Harvard University Press, 1986). Typical is the statement in Suleiman's introductory essay to the "Eros" section of this collection that, beginning with the new feminist movement in the 1970s, "the call went out to invent both a new poetics and a new politics, based on women's reclaiming what had always been theirs but had been usurped from them: control over their bodies and a voice with which to speak about it" (p. 7) and her description of the program of the French feminist Luce Irigaray: "To invent a language in which to speak about woman's pleasure and woman's love for woman — indeed, a language that will be addressed exclusively *to* women — this is, I think, the utopian ideal that Irigaray's text seeks both to project and in some approximate way to exemplify" (p. 14).

9.   Laura Mulvey, *Visual and Other Pleasures* (Bloomington and Indianapolis: Indiana University Press, 1989), pp. 16–17. Mulvey, in a series of essays written during the 1980s, gave the term "the male gaze" wide currency — particularly among feminist film critics, of which she is one. But the term (with its limiting assumptions) has become a commonplace of contemporary feminist criticism generally.

10.   John Berger's splendid 1972 essay on the history of portraiture of the female nude in the Western tradition, in *Ways of Seeing* (based on the BBC television series, London: British Broadcasting Corp. and Penguin Books, London, 1972, pp. 45–64) has been a particularly inspiring study for the present work. Not only did Berger analyze "the male gaze," and the interchange it implies between a male painter and a male spectator-purveyor about the woman's body which is its subject, long before the rest of us got there; he also understood, as few who have followed his lead have done, how an artist working within a convention can, through the way he manipulates his medium, transform its meaning — as Rubens, by painting his young wife in the act of turning, dispossesses the spectator, and turns a "sight" into an experience, an experience of tenderness and love, which the spectator is then invited to share.

See also John Beall's essay, "Gauguin's Uncanny Nude: Manao tupapau," *Rutgers Art Review* 11 (1990), pp. 37–51, and Wendy Lesser's recent study, *His Other Half: Men Looking at Women Through Art* (Cambridge, Mass. and London: Harvard University Press, 1991).

11. Carolyn G. Heilbrun, *Writing a Woman's Life* (New York: W. W. Norton, 1988). See p. 19 (on the dissemination of feminist ideas to "the general body of women"); see pp. 48ff. (on the possibilities of the "quest plot" for women).

12. "Visual impressions remain the most frequent pathway along which libidinal excitation is aroused; indeed, natural selection counts upon the accessibility of this pathway . . . when it encourages the development of beauty in the sexual object. The progressive concealment of the body which goes along with civilization keeps sexual curiosity awake. This curiosity seeks to complete the sexual object by revealing its hidden parts." And in a footnote to this essay Freud adds, "There is to my mind no doubt that the concept of 'beautiful' has its roots in sexual excitation and that its original meaning was 'sexually stimulating.'" *Three Essays on the Theory of Sexuality (1905*, footnote added 1915), vol. 7, in *The Standard Edition of the Psychological Works of Sigmund Freud*, 24 vols., trans. and ed. James Strachey (London: Hogarth Press and The Institute of Psychoanalysis, 1953), p. 156. See also the association Freud makes between the instincts for looking and for gaining knowledge, in *The General Theory of the Neuroses*, vol. 16, p. 327. On the splitting off of the passive desire for being looked at from the active desire for looking see *Instincts and Their Vicissitudes*, vol. 14, pp. 127–32. And on Freud's insistence that "the libido for looking and touching is present in everyone in two forms, active and passive . . . and, according to the preponderance of the sexual character, one form or the other predominates," see *Jokes and their Relation to the Unconscious*, vol. 8, p. 98.

13. Mulvey, *Visual*, p. 16 (my italics).

Chapter 2. *The Woman of Parts*

1. The story first makes its appearance in the Letters of Pliny the Elder in the first century A.D. (*Natural History*, 10 vols., with an English translation by H. Rackham, M.A. [Cambridge, Mass. and London: William Heinemann Limited, 1952], vol. 9, p. 309). Cicero (*De Inventore*, ii. I, I) is typical of the later tradition in assuming that Zeuxis took from each of the five maidens the best *part* of each to compose his ideal, but the story, as Pliny gives it to us, may simply mean that the artist availed himself of five different models the better to approximate the ideal of the one most beautiful woman. In the influential

Renaissance treatise by Agnolo Firenzuola, *Of the Beauty of Women*, trans. Clara Bell (London: McIlvaine & Company, 1892), we have a typical Renaissance elaboration of the story: the artist moderates a dispute among four women about the beauty of a fifth by tactfully announcing that, in the manner of Zeuxis, he will take the best part of each of them to compose his ideally beautiful woman (p. 30).

2.   Sir Walter Scott, *Ivanhoe* (New York: Signet, New American Library, 1962), chap. 2, pp. 46–47. All subsequent quotations are from this edition.

3.   So John Suckling introduces his portrait of the rustic bride in "A Ballad Upon a Wedding," with the fraternal overture, "I'll tell thee, *Dick*, where I have béen, / Where I the rarest things have seen; / Oh things without compare!" *The Norton Anthology of Poetry*, 3d ed., ed. Alexander W. Allison, *et al.* (New York and London: W. W. Norton, 1983), p. 319. Nancy Vickers, in an article on Shakespeare's long dramatic poem, *The Rape of Lucrece*, suggests that the real impetus behind the catalogue portrait of the beautiful woman is not any feelings for the woman but rivalry between men. "This Heraldray in Lucrece' Face," originally published in *Poetics Today* 6 (1985), reprinted in *The Female Body in Western Culture: Contemporary Perspectives*, ed. Susan Rubin Suleiman (Cambridge: Harvard University Press, 1986), pp. 209–22.

4.   Rowena's situation is made graphic in Robert Browning's famous poem, "My Last Duchess," where the two men, host and guest, stand not before the woman herself as they appraise her but before her literally immobilized figure: her portrait on the wall. In the stunning last lines of Browning's poem we are made to realize (as not in Scott) the killing effect of such masculine appropriation of the woman's body. She was his *"last* Duchess," and his treatment of her during her lifetime as an art object has been the death of the real woman.

5.   "Criticism of Female Beauty" (c. 1850), in Leigh Hunt, *Men, Women, and Books; a Selection of Sketches, Essays, and Critical Memoirs, from his Uncollected Prose Writings* (London: Smith, Elder, 1847), p. 249.

6.   See Nancy J. Vickers, "Diana Described: Scattered Woman and Scattered Rhyme," in *Writing and Sexual Difference*, ed. Elizabeth Abel (Chicago: University of Chicago Press, 1980), pp. 95–109, for an interesting discussion of Petrarchan dismemberment. Vickers does not, however, make a distinction between the two kinds of "partial" seeing, and views Petrarchan dismemberment as the primary model for the later tradition of patriarchal heroine-portraiture.

7.   "Physical beauty arises from the harmonious effect of manifold parts that can be taken in at one view. It demands also that these parts shall subsist side

by side; and as things whose parts subsist side by side are the proper subject of painting, so it, and it alone, can imitate physical beauty. The poet, who can only show the elements of beauty one after another, in succession, does on that very account forbear altogether the description of physical beauty, as beauty. He recognizes that those elements, arranged in succession, cannot possibly have the effect which they have when placed side by side; that the concentrating gaze which we would direct upon them immediately after their enumeration still affords us no harmonious picture." Lessing, *Laocoön; Nathan the Wise; Minna von Barnhelm*, ed. William A. Steel (London: J. M. Dent & Sons Limited, 1930), sec. 20, p. 74.

8.   *Orlando Furioso*, 1532, Canto 7, st. 14, in *Selections from the Translation of Sir John Harrington*, ed. Rudolf Gottfried (Bloomington: Indiana University Press, 1963), p. 155.

9.   *The Complete Poetry of John Donne*, with an Introduction, notes, and variants by John T. Shawcross (New York and London: New York University Press and University of London Press, Limited, 1968), ll. 25–27, p. 58.

10.   *The Elegies of Maximian*, ed. Richard Webster (Princeton: Princeton University Press, 1900), Elegy I, ll. 93–99, p. 13. I translate: "The long golden hair and the neck like new poured milk; / The large guiless features which adorned her noble face; / The black eyebrows; the broad forehead; the bright eye: / All these, often noted, burned my soul. / I loved the flaming red and slightly swelling lips — / The kind from which I have been granted many delightful kisses."

11.   On the history and probable sources of the convention which appears fully developed in the French romances of the late twelfth and thirteenth centuries see the following discussions. Edmond Faral cites Maximian's Elegy I as the earliest example of the conventional portrait of the ideally beautiful woman, in *Les Arts poétiques du XIIͤ et du XIIIͤ siècle*, Bibliotèque de l'Ecole des Hautes Etudes, no. 238 (Paris: Champion, 1924), pp. 80–81. Edgar de Bruyne stresses the codification of the convention by the twelfth-century rhetoricians Matthew of Vendôme and Geoffrey of Vinsauf (see my discussion on pp. 42–44) and suggests that already by the twelfth century there is some expression of weariness with the conventional epithets, in *Etudes d'esthétique médiévale* (Geneva: Slatkine Reprints, 1975), vol. 2, *L'Epoque romane*, bk. 3, chap. 4, sec. 3. "Amour ou mépris de la beauté féminine," pp. 173–202. D. S. Brewer sees in the fifth-century Dares Phrygius "the late-Classical ideal of feminine beauty ready to receive its medieval development," but also cites Maximian's elegy as "establish[ing] the type to which *every* lady conforms in all the medieval Latin and vernacular literature of Europe," in "The Ideal of

Feminine Beauty in Medieval Literature, Especially 'Harley Lyrics,' Chaucer, and Some Elizabethans," *Modern Language Review* 50 (1955), pp. 257 and 258. Peter Dronke rightly observes that Maximian's elegy does not really particularize the features of the beautiful woman, and is rather in the tradition of the lament for the lost beauty of the world than that of "descriptio" *per se*. Dronke cites earlier poems of classical and Christian antiquity (by Claudian and Venantius Fortunatus, respectively) in which we find elements of the catalogue and some of the recurrent similes of the later convention, in *Medieval Latin and the Rise of the European Love Lyric*, 2 vols. (Oxford: Clarendon Press, 1965), vol. 1, p. 195.

12.   See Paul Salmon, "The Wild Man in 'Iwein' and Medieval Descriptive Technique," *Modern Language Review* 56, no. 4 (Oct. 1961), pp. 520–28.

13.   Geoffrey of Vinsauf, *Poetria Nova*, trans. Margaret F. Nims (Toronto: Pontifical Institute of Medieval Studies, 1967), pp. 36–37. All of the quotations which follow are from these pages. De Bruyne, *Etudes*, and Brewer, "Ideal," both stress the importance of the twelfth-century rhetoricians (Matthew and Geoffrey) in codifying — and rigidifying — for the later tradition the practice of earlier poets. Classical rhetoricians have little to say about descriptive techniques. Cicero explicitly cautions that the accidentals of appearance are irrelevant to the poet's praise (*De Oratore*, bk. 2, 84. 342). Priscian in the fifth century A.D. advises the poet, when praising a hero, to note how strong he is in body, how large in size, how excellent in soul, how just, how wise, how temperate, etc., in *Rhetores Latini Minores*, ed. C. Halm (Leipzig: B. G. Teubner, 1863), "Prisciani Grammatici" and "De Laude," p. 556, which hardly constitutes encouragement for a descriptive catalogue. An important authority for the classification of the art of description ("descriptio") — as a branch of epidictic poetry, the purpose of which is to hold up an individual for praise or blame — is the *Ad Herennium*, a rhetorical treatise of late antiquity but believed in the Middle Ages to be Cicero's. "Descriptio" is divided into two types, of character ("notatio") and physical ("effictio"). "Effictio" itself is then divided, e.g., in Matthew of Vendôme (see below), into two branches — affirmative (for descriptions of the ideally beautiful body) and negative (for descriptions of the ideally ugly body). See the discussion of "Descriptio" in Ernest Gallo, *The "Poetria Nova" and Its Sources in Early Rhetorical Doctrine* (The Hague and Paris: Mouton, 1971), pp. 177–87.

14.   See the top-to-toe portrait of the goddess Nature in Alan of Lille's late twelfth-century poem, *The Plaint of Nature* (*De Planctu Naturae*), where the narrator observes, at the same critical juncture, that "faith spoke other parts, which a more secret habitation held aside, to be even better" (282A–87); II,

Prose 1; *The Plaint of Nature*, trans. James J. Sheridan (Toronto: Pontifical Institute of Mediaeval Studies, 1980). The thirteenth-century rhetorician, Brunetto Latini, concludes an exemplary portrait of the beautiful woman with the words: "But I shall remain silent about the other parts of her body, of which the heart can speak better than the tongue." James R. East, *Book III of Brunetto Latini's Tresor: An English Translation and Assessment of its Contribution to Rhetorical Theory* (Ph.D. dissertation, Stanford University, 1960), p. 123. Matthew of Vendôme (see discussion below), drawing upon the evaluative vocabulary of the convention in a portrait of Helen of Troy, says, "The sweetness of savor that lies hid in the realm of Venus / The *judging* touch can foretell," *Ars Versificatoria (The Art of the Verse Maker)*, trans. Roger P. Parr (Milwaukee: Marquette University Press, 1981), sec. 57, p. 38 (my italics).

15.   Donne, *Complete Poetry*, 1. 89, p. 67.

16.   Alice M. Colby, *The Portrait in Twelfth-Century French Literature: An Example of the Stylistic Originality of Chrétien de Troyes* (Geneva: Librairie Droz, 1965), p. 62.

17.   My translation. The French text reads: "K'en dites vus de cel desuz / Ke nus apelum le cunet? Je quit qe asez fut petitet." *Ipomédon, poème de Hué de Rotélande*, ed. J. Holden (Paris: Editions Kincksieck, 1979), ll. 2268–70, p. 167.

18.   Matthew of Vendôme, *Ars Versificatoria*, sec. 58, p. 39. All subsequent quotations are from this text.

19.   Christopher Marlowe, *The Complete Poems and Translations*, ed. Stephen Orgel (Harmondsworth, England: Penguin, 1971), sestiad I, ll. 61–69, p. 19.

20.   Henry Fielding, *Joseph Andrews*, "preceded by" *Shamela*, ed. A. R. Humphreys (London and New York: Dent & Dutton, 1973), bk. 1, chap. 8, pp. 18–19).

21.   Sidonius Apollinarus' mid-fifth-century A.D. portrait of the Emperor Theodoric, recommended by Geoffrey of Vinsauf in his second rhetorical treatise, the *Documentum* (II. 2. 10), as a model for portraitists working in prose, is an interesting example of a male subject who, while laid out for us in top-to-toe sequence, refuses to "sit (or to lie) still" for his portrait. See Sidonius Apollinarus, *Poems and Letters*, ed. and trans. W. B. Anderson, 2 vols. (Cambridge: Harvard University Press, 1936), "To Agricola," vol. 1, bk. 1, letter 2, pp. 335–37.

22.   Blanche, whose death is mourned fulsomely in *The Book of the Duchess*, receives Chaucer's most extensive and conventional portrait. In *Troilus and Criseyde*, where the tripartite panel of portraits of the three leading characters, Criseyde, Troilus, and his rival, Diomede (bk. V, ll. 799–840), might encour-

age us to expect symmetry, there is much more attention to Criseyde's physical appearances than to the men who frame her on either side.

23.   I am pursuing a line of argument here suggested by my reading of Quen-
tin Bell's fascinating study of changing fashions in dress, *On Human Finery* (2d
ed. New York: Schocken Books, 1976). Drawing on Thorstein Veblen's famous analysis of the theory of the leisure class, Bell points out that in the postindustrial world, where wealth is based on capital assets rather than land ownership and even wealthy men assume the uniform dress of the "worker," their
wives continue to display the elegant, constricting clothing that testifies to
their husbands' wealth: the women wear on their backs, so to speak, the em-
blems of their husbands' success. I would add that the shift in the language
used to describe the bodies *inside* the clothing, which occurs contemporane-
ously, sends out the same message of differentiation by sex rather than by
class — with perhaps even greater force.

     Colby (in *Portrait*) stresses the fact that the twelfth-century French romanc-
ers not only confer similar physical features on their heroes and heroines but
employ essentially the same formal devices: particularly the top-to-toe catalogue of parts. She does note, however, that there are fewer such portraits of
heroes than of heroines in the romances (ten altogether laudatory portraits of
men as compared with twenty-two of heroines) and that the masculine portraits are somewhat shorter than their female counterparts (an average of
forty-five lines for the men as compared to forty-nine for the women — this
last, to be sure, not a very significant difference). What we see in the rhetorical
treatises is neater than what we see in the romances themselves: perhaps it
takes time for practice to "catch up with" theory.

24.   In the French romances the same term ("bel" for the man, "belle" for the
woman) is applied to both sexes. In 1811 Jane Austen can still refer to the
"manly beauty" of Mr. Willoughby (in *Sense and Sensibility*, with an afterword by Caroline Mercer [New York: Penguin, Signet, 1980], vol. 1, chap.
9, p. 37). It is perhaps relevant, however, that this introductory description
comes to us from the public voice, and Willoughby is eventually discovered
by the novel's heroine to be something less than an ideally "manly man."

25.   On the medieval convention of heroine portraiture see the various ex-
amples cited in Colby, *Portrait*. In Chrétien de Troyes, the greatest of the
twelfth-century romancers, see particularly the top-to-toe portrait of "The
Ugly Maiden," ll. 4610–37, in *Percival, or, The Story of the Grail*, trans. Ruth
Harwood Cline (New York: Pergamon Press, 1983). See also *Aucassin and Ni-
colette*, a French romance of the thirteenth century, in which the hero's portrait
is very abbreviated compared to the heroine's (pp. 13–14), in *Aucassin & Ni-*

colette and other Medieval Romances and Legends, trans. Eugene Mason (London: J. M. Dent & Sons, Limited, 1910), pp. 1–2. And see my discussion of Chaucer above and in n. 21.

26. Of the many extended Renaissance portraits, my own list of the most notable includes the following: Spenser's portrait of his own virtuous bride in the *Epithalamion* (1589), where having descended in the usual progression downward from eyes, cheeks, lips, breast, "and all her body like a pallace fayre," the poet-lover reverses his direction, and "ascend[s] vppe with many a stately stayre, / To honors seat and chastities sweet bowre," in *The Poetical Works of Edmund Spenser,* vol. 1, *Spenser's Minor Poems,* ed. Ernest de Sélincourt (Oxford: Clarendon Press, 1960), pp. 426–27, ll. 179–80; Ariosto's exuberant and lengthy portrait of Alcina in the *Orlando Furioso* (1532), Canto 7, stanzas 10–15, in Gottfried, *Harrington,* pp. 154–55; Tasso's portrait of the enchantress Armida in the *Gerusalemme Liberata* (1557), Canto 4, stanzas 29–32, which says that though her robe "to the eyes . . . closes the path" to her breast, "it does not wholly check the amorous mind, which — being not well content with outward beauty — works itself still within to the hidden secrets," in Torquato Tasso, *Jerusalem Delivered. An English Prose Version,* trans. and ed. Ralph Nash (Detroit: Wayne State University Press, 1987), stanza 31, p. 75; and Thomas Lodge's portrait of Scilla, in his 1589 romance, *Scillaes Metamorphosis,* where, as in Donne's "Loves Progress," the poet's downward progression with his eyes is explicitly joined to the lover's descent toward his place of greatest good, in *The Complete Works of Thomas Lodge* (New York: Russell & Russell, 1963), vol. 1, "Glaucus and Scilla," pp. 14–15.

27. See particularly the portrait of Sophia in *Tom Jones* (1749), one of the most exuberant and most extended of later-day instances. Typically of Fielding, this one is part parody and part the real thing (bk. 4, chap. 2, "A short Hint of what we can do in the Sublime, and a Description of Miss Sophia Western.") *The History of Tom Jones: A Foundling,* ed. Sheridan Baker (New York: W. W. Norton, 1973), pp. 116–18.

28. A particularly interesting mid-Victorian example of the convention is the portrait of Laura Bell in Thackeray's *Pendennis* (1848–50), where we get almost no details of the heroine's appearance on our first sight of her at the opening of the novel. But that is because Arthur Pendennis is still philandering about and doesn't know enough to take proper cognizance of her. Laura's elevation to heroine status, about one-third of the way through the novel, is signaled by the fact that the author now arrests the flow of his narrative to take her picture — despite his prefatory disclaimer that he is "not good at descriptions of female beauty; and, indeed, do[es] not care for it in the least (thinking

that goodness and virtue are, of course, far more advantageous to a young lady than any mere fleeting charms of person and face) . . ." (bk. 1, chap. 21). We know exactly what to expect: the page and a half of feature-by-feature evaluation which follows.

29.   Laurence Sterne, *The Life and Opinions of Tristram Shandy, Gentleman*, ed. James Aiken Work (New York: Odyssey Press, 1940), pp. 469–71.

30.   James Joyce, *A Portrait of the Artist as a Young Man* (New York: Viking, 1969), p. 171.

31.   Vladimir Nabokov, *Lolita* (New York: Perigee Books, 1980), p. 39.

32.   Samuel Richardson, *Clarissa: Or the History of a Young Lady* (1748), ed. John Angus Burrell (New York: Random House, 1950), "Mr. Lovelace to John Belford, Esq.," Tuesday, Wedn., April 11, 12, pp. 221–22. All subsequent quotations are from this edition.

Chapter 3. *Beauty and Identity*

1.   The heroines of the popular late-eighteenth-century novelist, Ann Radcliffe, for instance, are typical "fairest maids." And in the nineteenth century, particularly in second-rate women's fiction, the inventory of the heroine's beautiful parts continues to flourish. Mrs. Marsh's Emilia Wyndam, a heroine held up for contrast by one reviewer with her contemporary, Jane Eyre, has "two very expressive eyes of whatever colour you please to call them, for no one could ever decide the matter—a sweet, delicate mouth, expressive of both sense, temper and feeling—a nice, steady round chin—abundance of brown hair, a colour like a rose—a light, elastic, but somewhat full-formed figure, with a pair of the most beautiful arms in the world, which last advantage gave a singular elegance to her gestures," to which inventory is appended the standard proviso: "However when you were with her, or talking to her, you seemed as little to think of what she looked like as she did herself" (*Emilia Wyndam*, by the author of *Two Old Men's Tales, Mount Sorrel*, etc. [Paris: Galignani, 1846], chap. 1, p. 11). Maria Edgeworth, the great Irish novelist of the late eighteenth and nineteenth centuries (who makes frequent references to her sense of her own personal unattractiveness in her letters) never creates a heroine whose beauty is in any sense questionable. Edgeworth does, however, at times point ironically to the conventionality of her own practice—as when the witty younger sister of the lovely Caroline, heroine of *Patronage* (1814), declares with at least a touch of asperity at the novel's opening that any available suitors will inevitably be drawn to her sister, with "superior claims

of every sort, and with that most undisputed of all the rights of woman —
beauty" — as indeed they are. Maria Edgeworth, *Patronage*, 4 vols. (London:
J. J. Johnson & Company, 1814), vol. 1, p. 2. The practice of Fanny Burney,
whose published fiction spans the critical years between 1778 and 1814, gives
us a nice index of how heroine-portraiture changes in the work of a major
woman novelist. Thus the beauty of her first heroine is "so striking, it is not
possible to pass it unnoticed" (*Evelina, or the History of a Young Lady's Entrance
into the World*, ed. Edward A. Bloom with the assistance of Lillian D. Bloom
[Oxford and New York: Oxford University Press, 1982], vol. 1, letter 6, p.
21. Cecilia's beauty (in 1782) is no less striking, but now each beautiful feature
of her face "announces" a beauty within. Camilla, in 1796, is a classic "difficult" beauty, set off by her rivalry with a "picture-book" beauty drawn in the
old style (see my discussion below, pp. 69–70). Juliet, the heroine of Burney's
last novel, *The Wanderer* (1814), seems, at first blush, to take us even farther:
when first seen, her aspect, as her identity, is shrouded in mystery. Yet, to my
mind at least, underneath her "black-face" disguise and the camouflage of her
dress, Juliet turns out to be as disappointingly conventional in spirit as she is
in the revealed red-and-white of her fair complexion. To generalize (perhaps
to over-generalize): the greatest male novelists, even into our own age, like
Scott in the nineteenth century, continue to portray their heroines in the evaluative terms of the patriarchal convention; the greatest women novelists, by
the early nineteenth century, are reinventing that convention.

2. I have found particularly useful in researching the earlier, less well known
women novelists Jane Spencer's compelling and beautifully nuanced study,
The Rise of the Woman Novelist from Aphra Behn to Jane Austen (Oxford and
New York: B. Blackwell, 1986). Spencer is more sanguine than some other
recent feminists about the ability of women writers in this (and in later) pe-
riods to shape the instruments of masculine discourse to the purposes of their
own speech.

3. Woolf, *A Room of One's Own and Three Guineas*, with an Introduction by
Hermione Lee (London: Chatto & Windus, Hogarth Press, 1984), p. 84.

4. Fanny Burney, *Camilla, or A Picture of Youth*, ed. with an Introduction by
Edward A. Bloom and Lillian D. Bloom (Oxford and New York: Oxford
University Press, 1983), vol. 1, bk. 1, chap. 2, p. 22. All subsequent quota-
tions are from this edition.

5. Samuel Johnson, *The Rambler*, ed. W. J. Bate and Albrecht B. Strauss,
3 vols. (New Haven and London: Yale University Press, 1969), vol. 2, pp.
344–45.

6.   The author of this *Spectator* essay (no. 17, March 20, 1711) is in fact Steele, not Addison. Where Johnson's inflections are grave, Steele expounds the same moral in a lighter, even jocular, vein: "Since our Persons are not of our own making, when they are such as appear Defective or Uncomely, it is, methinks, an honest and laudable Fortitude to dare to be Ugly; at least to keep ourselves from being abashed with a Consciousness of Imperfection which we cannot help, and in which there is no Guilt. I would not defend [i.e., condemn] an haggard Beau, for passing away much time at a Glass, and giving Softness and Languishing Graces to Deformity. All I intend is, that we ought to be contented with our Countenance and Shape, so far, as never to give ourselves an uneasie Reflection on that Subject." See also *Spectator*, nos. 33, 144, and 306 (April 7, 1711; August 15, 1711; and February 20, 1712).

7.   There is an interesting reading of this episode in Margaret Doody's biography of Fanny Burney, *Frances Burney: The Life in the Works* (New Brunswick: Rutgers University Press, 1988). Doody points out that the Reverend Tyrold — who underlines his moral by forcing Eugenia to play the part of the spectator to the sight of an imprisoned, beautiful-but-mad woman so that she may appreciate the superiority of her own "inner beauty" — is reenacting the recent scene of Eugenia's own humiliation, where she was imprisoned to be gazed at by the market-women. Thus, her father "has merely mechanically repeated the turning of the female into a spectacle, the being to be observed, not heard" (pp. 229–30).

8.   After teasing us all the way through *Bleak House* with the question of Esther Summerson's disfigurement after her contagion (mirrors are removed, a former suitor makes an awkward retreat, and perhaps most significantly, from the reader's point of view, in all the illustrations in which Esther appears *after* her disease we are only allowed to see her from the back or with her face obscured), Esther's worthy husband tells her on the novel's very last page ("didn't she know?") she is prettier than she ever was — which Esther, of course, won't believe, because both she herself and those who love her "can very well do without much beauty in me — even supposing — " (Charles Dickens, *Bleak House*, ed. George Ford and Sylvère Monod [New York: W. W. Norton, 1977], chap. 67, p. 770). Dickens's tease here is a wonderfully effective one; but it differs from what we see more typically in women's fiction precisely because it *is* such a tease: we know all along how much Esther's beauty matters, and our curiosity is only intensified by her insistence throughout that it *doesn't* matter. *Bleak House*, which is Dickens's only novel to employ a female narrative voice, is also his only experiment in the difficult beauty convention (Esther has her foil in the conventionally beautiful Ada), and it is a

characteristically Dickensian experiment. For Dickens's general style of heroine-portraiture in his fiction see n. 31 below.

9. *Cœlebs in Search of a Wife: Comprehending Observations on Domestic Habits and Manners, Religion and Morals*, 2 vols. (London: T. Cadwell & W. Davies, 1809), vol. 1, chap. 14, pp. 185–86.

10. The *Oxford English Dictionary* does not mark the sense I am defining here, but rather distinguishes between two usages which, it notes, are not always easy to separate from one another in practice — namely: countenance as "the outer, ever-changing expression on the face," as in "a man's countenance varies; his face is always the same" (1859, *OED*, 2d ed., 4); and countenance as "the appearance of the face, the tablet on which the emotions may come and go," as in "How hope succeeds despair on each captain's countenance" (1871, *OED* 5). It is true that "countenance" can span the full range of possibilities between these two poles. But I think a third, intermediate sense is often clearly indicated, in which "countenance" is defined, as in the instances I cite here, as the more or less permanent record laid down on our features by habitual thoughts and feelings.

11. In a 1771 letter by Benjamin Franklin, "countenance" is the pivotal term for a definition of beauty which comes about as close as anything I have seen to defining beauty as I would define it — as the emerging face of love. Writing to the mother of his young godson, and detailing his prescription for the proper rearing of the child, Franklin notes that a happy childhood (and for him that means essentially an unconstrained one) will leave a lasting mark on an individual's appearance: "Pray let him have every thing he likes," Franklin dictates. "I think it of great Consequence while the Features of the *Countenance* are forming. It gives them a pleasant Air, and that being once become natural, and fix'd by Habit, the Face is ever the handsomer for it, and on that much of a Person's good Fortune and Success in Life may depend" (*The Papers of Benjamin Franklin*, 30 vols., ed. W. B. Wilcox [New Haven: Yale University Press, 1959–], vol. 18, pp. 252–53). Franklin nicely pays tribute here to the role of appearances in determining the individual's later happiness in life, while at the same time implying that beauty is not a privilege but (as the consequence of an education guided by libertarian principles) one of the individual's natural rights.

12. Elizabeth Inchbald, *A Simple Story*, ed. J. M. S. Tompkins (London: Oxford University Press, 1967), chap. 2, p. 12.

13. Jane Austen, *Pride and Prejudice*, with an Afterword by Joann Morse (New York: Signet, New American Library, 1980), vol. 1, chap. 3, p. 12. All subsequent quotations are from this edition.

14.   *OED*, 2d ed., "pretty" I. For "pretty" in later usages see the following *OED* notations: 2.a. "of persons — clever skillful, apt"; 3.a. "having a proper appearance, brave, gallant, stout warlike" (cites "pretty fellow"); 4. "having beauty without majesty or stateliness; beautiful in a slight, dainty, or diminutive way, as opposed to *handsome*."

15.   *OED*, 2d ed. The following *OED* citations for "handsome" are particularly relevant here: 1.a. "easy to handle" (obs.); 4.a. "of fair size"; 4.b. "of a sum of money, ample, generous, munificent." So Austen's "handsome" woman is herself a large (if not perhaps ultimately desirable) object up for sale.

16.   Nabokov, *Lolita*, p. 74.

17.   The complacency of the "handsome" woman is established in Austen's very early juvenilia, where the heroine of her epistolary farce *Lesley Castle* (written when she was seventeen years old) writes, "We are handsome, my dear Charlotte, very handsome, and the greatest of our Perfections is, that we are entirely insensible of them." *Lesley Castle: An Unfinished Novel in Letters*, in *Love and Freindship* [sic] *and other Early Works*, with a preface by G. K. Chesterton (New York: Frederick A. Stokes Company, 1920), p. 59.

18.   Jane Austen, *Northanger Abbey*, with an Afterword by Elizabeth Hardwick (New York: Signet, New American Library, 1980), chap. 4, p. 25.

19.   Jane Austen, *Mansfield Park*, with an Afterword by Marvin Mudrick (New York: Signet, New American Library, 1979), vol. 1, chap. 5, p. 37. All subsequent quotations are from this edition.

20.   Jane Austen, *Persuasion*, with an Afterword by Marvin Mudrick (New York: Signet, New American Library, 1980), vol. 1, chap. 1, p. 12. All subsequent quotations are from this edition.

21.   In *The Watsons*, there is an echo of the Elizabeth-Jane Bennet contrast: "Many were the eyes, and various the degrees of approbation with which [Emma] was examined. Some saw no fault, and some no beauty. With some her brown skin was the annihilation of every grace, and others could never be persuaded that she were *half so handsome* as Elizabeth Watson had been ten years ago" (my italics). In Jane Austen, *Lady Susan, The Watsons, Sanditon*, ed. with an Introduction by Margaret Drabble (Harmondsworth, England: Penguin, 1974), pp. 128–29. And finally, in Austen's last, unfinished fragment, *Sanditon*, the emergent beauty of the heroine, Charlotte, is played off against the spectacle of an old-convention handsome young woman as Charlotte first sees her: "Elegantly tall, regularly handsome, with great delicacy of complexion and soft blue eyes, a sweetly modest and yet naturally graceful address,

Charlotte could see in her only the most perfect representation of whatever heroine might be most beautiful and bewitching, in all the numerous volumes they had left behind them on Mrs Whitby's shelves." Ibid., p. 179.

22. *The Life of Mary Russell Mitford, Told by Herself in Letters to Her Friends,* ed. the Rev. A. G. K. L'Estrange, 2 vols. (New York: Harper & Brothers, 1870), vol. 1, chap. 9, p. 235.

23. These reminiscences come to us second-hand, from Mrs. Harriet Mozley's letter of 2 November 1838, giving Fulwar William Fowle's description of the impression made on him by the young Jane Austen at the country dances which were her greatest delight. My source is Park Honan, *Jane Austen: Her Life* (New York: Fawcett Columbine, Ballantine Books, 1987), p. 87.

24. In *Jane Austen's Letters to her Sister Cassandra and Others,* collected and ed. R. W. Chapman, 2 vols. (Oxford: Clarendon Press, 1932), vol. 2, letter 91, p. 371.

25. Samuel Richardson, *Pamela: Or Virtue Rewarded* (New York: W. W. Norton, 1958), letter 2, p. 5. All subsequent quotations are from this edition.

26. Pamela's letters are no longer numbered.

27. Elizabeth Gaskell, *North and South,* with an Introduction by Martin Dodsworth (Harmondsworth, England: Penguin, 1970), p. 35.

28. Harriet Martineau, *Deerbrook,* with a new Introduction by Gaby Weiner (London: Virago Press Limited, 1983), p. 6.

29. Mrs. Oliphant, *Kirsteen,* with an Introduction by Merryn Williams (London: Dent, 1984), p. 3.

30. Jeanne Fahnestock, in "The Heroine of Irregular Features, Physiognomy and Conventions of Heroine Description," *Victorian Studies* (Spring, 1981), pp. 325–50, sees many of the same features I am noting here but interprets them in terms of novelists' increasing command of realistic detail. Along somewhat similar lines, Michael Irwin, in *Picturing: Description and Illusion in the Nineteenth Century Novel* (London: George Allen & Unwin, Limited, 1979), analyzes descriptive techniques in terms of their value as indicators of character.

31. Dickens's heroine-portraiture deserves a study of its own. He consistently repudiates the patriarchal convention, as it is perpetuated in nineteenth-century male fiction, particularly by his great compeer Thackeray. But Dickens has his own way of making the sexuality of his heroines into something safe. He does not inventory their assets but gives them the blurred outlines

through which they might be seen by the eye of childhood. The "littleness" which is the salient physical feature of Dickens's heroines (from Little Nell to Little Em'ly to Little Dorrit) does not imply a larger, commanding masculine observer. His childlike heroine is often at the same time the protecting mother, just as the male observer through whose loving gaze we see her is himself both parent and child. For the world in which the Dickensian hero and heroine may find a temporary refuge is the undifferentiated paradise of infancy. Thus the apotheosis of the Dickensian heroine is when the beautiful but bad Bella Wilfer ("the lovely woman") in Dickens's last completed novel, is appropriately re-christened as a mark of her transformation into a good woman, by the poor boy Johnny in his dying breath as "the boofer lady." *Our Mutual Friend*, with an Introduction by E. Salter Davies (New York and Oxford: Oxford University Press, 1991), bk. 2, chap. 9, p. 330.

32.   *The Warden*, with an Introduction and notes by David Skilton (World Classics éd., Oxford and New York: Oxford University Press, 1980), p. 139.

33.   Edmund Burke, *A Philosophical Enquiry into the Origin of our Ideas of the Sublime and Beautiful*, ed. James T. Boulton (Notre Dame and London: University of Notre Dame Press, 1968), sec. 16, p. 116.

34.   See Bettelheim's, *The Uses of Enchantment: The Meaning and Importance of Fairy Tales* (New York: Vintage, 1977). I have drawn upon Bettelheim's wonderful reading of *Cinderella* (pp. 236–77) here — though not for my analysis of the tale's concluding affirmation.

35.   See the interesting study by Huang Mei, *Transforming the Cinderella Dream: From Frances Burney to Charlotte Bronte* (New Brunswick and London: Rutgers University Press, 1990), which suggests that Cinderella, a more active heroine than Sleeping Beauty or Snow White, emblemizes a tension between an ideal of humility and that of aspiration — both traits for which, like the typical nineteenth-century English heroine, she is rewarded.

36.   Bettelheim, *Uses of Enchantment*, pp. 250ff. See also Marian R. Cox, *Cinderella: Three Hundred and Forty-five Variants* (London: David Nutt, 1893).

37.   "Ashputtle," in *Grimm's Tales for Young and Old*, trans. Ralph Manheim (New York: Doubleday & Company, Inc., 1977, Anchor Books, 1983), p. 85.

38.   Bettelheim enforces the importance of an affirmation of Cinderella's identity at the end of the story, though in somewhat different terms than mine — seeing it as the acceptance of the bad as well as the good aspects of her nature, "because any true identity has its negative as well as its positive as-

pects" (p. 275). He also notes that in variant versions of *Cinderella* it is clear that an oedipal attachment to her father is the explanation for Cinderella's present degradation and provides a real basis for her own conviction of being, at least in part, a bad child. In this sense, the fairy tale might be said to go further than Burney's latter-day fiction.

39.   The closest Austen ever comes to an objective appraisal is when she says of Marianne Dashwood in *Sense and Sensibility*, that "when in the common cant of praise she was called a beautiful girl, truth was less violently outraged than usually happens." *Sense and Sensibility*, with an Afterword by Caroline Mercer (New York: Penguin, Signet, 1980), vol. 1, chap. 10, p. 40.

40.   See the frequent references to Jane's conspicuously rosy cheeks in her youth, for example, by Egerton Brydges, quoted in J. E. Austen-Leigh, *A Memoir of Jane Austen* (2d ed., London: Bentley, 1871), p. 48; quoted in Honan, *Jane Austen*, p. 61. Honan also quotes an excerpt from a burlesque Austen wrote at the age of fourteen in which she parodies those same rosy cheeks, insisting (when accused of drunkenness), "I deny that it is possible for anyone to have too great a proportion of red in their cheeks" (p. 71).

41.   Elizabeth Gaskell, *Wives and Daughters*, ed. Frank Glover Smith (Harmondsworth, England: Penguin, 1969), chap. 13, p. 187.

42.   Hans Christian Andersen, *Andersen's Fairy Tales*, trans. Pat Shaw Iversen (New York: Penguin, Signet, 1987), p. 137. All subsequent quotations are from this edition.

43.   Margaret Drabble, *A Summer Bird-Cage* (Harmondsworth, England: Penguin, 1967), chap. 2, p. 21. All subsequent quotations are from this edition.

Chapter 4. *Charlotte Brontë*

1.   From Ellen Nussey's first impressions of the fourteen-year-old Charlotte Brontë at the Roe Head school: in *The Brontës: Their Lives, Friendships and Correspondence*, 4 vols., ed. Thomas J. Wise and J. A. Symington (Oxford: Basil Blackwell, 1932), vol. 1, p. 92. This source hereafter referred to as *SHBLL* (The Shakespeare Head Brontë).

2.   George Lewes's impression on meeting "Currer Bell," as reported by George Eliot in a letter to the Brays, in *The George Eliot Letters*, 9 vols., ed. Gordon S. Haight (New Haven: Yale University Press, 1954–78), vol. 2, p. 91.

3. George Murray Smith, "Charlotte Brontë," *Cornhill Magazine* 82 (December 1900).

4. Lady Amberly, a free-thinking noblewoman who defied convention by accompanying her husband to visit George Eliot in 1867 (in *Amberly Papers* [2 vols., 1937], vol. 2, p. 58; quoted in Gordon S. Haight, *George Eliot: A Biography* (1968; London: Penguin, 1985), p. 391.

5. The eminent American scholar Charles Eliot Norton in letter to G. W. Curtis, 29 January 1869 (manuscript at Harvard) published in Haight, *Letters*, vol. 5, pp. 8–9.

6. The young Henry James, after his first meeting with the then-famous novelist in 1869, in a letter to his father (10 May 1869) in Henry James, *Selected Letters*, ed. Leon Edel (Cambridge, Mass.: Belknap Press of Harvard University Press, 1987), p. 35.

7. Pickering, *Creative Malady: Illness in the Lives and Minds of Charles Darwin, Florence Nightingale, Mary Baker Eddy, Sigmund Freud, Marcel Proust, and Elizabeth Barrett Browning* (London: George Allen & Unwin, Limited, 1974).

8. *SHBLL*, vol. 4, p. 203.

9. As reported to her friend Harriet Martineau, and quoted in turn in the latter's obituary of Brontë in *The Daily News*, April 1855; reprinted in *SHBLL*, vol. 4, p. 180.

10. *Jane Eyre*, ed. Q. D. Leavis (London and New York: Viking-Pengin, 1985), chap. 10, p. 122. All subsequent quotations are from this edition.

11. As reported to her friend Harriet Martineau, and quoted in turn in the latter's obituary of Brontë in *The Daily News*, April 1855; reprinted in *SHBLL*, vol. 4, p. 180.

12. Elizabeth Rigby (Lady Eastlake), *The Quarterly Review* 90 (1851), pp. 62–91. Although Rigby suggests that it is "a woman's *business* to be beautiful," in categorizing the various orders of beauty (and particularly in distinguishing the English ideal from the French), she says that the highest order of beauty is not that of coloring or feature but of expression — or countenance: her own ideal is thus, in its own way, a version of the "difficult" beauty.

13. *The Quarterly Review* 87 (December 1848), p. 167.

14. Bagehot, "The Waverly Novels," in *Literary Studies*, ed. Richard Holt Hutton, 2 vols. (London: Longmans, Green & Company, 1879), vol. 2,

p. 167. These essays are republished papers first written for the *National Review*. On the vogue for the plain heroine, inspired by *Jane Eyre*, see Kathleen Tillotson, *Novels of the Eighteen-Forties* (Oxford: Oxford University Press, 1983), p. 260, n. 2; and Patricia Thomson, *The Victorian Heroine: A Changing Ideal* (Oxford: Oxford University Press, 1956), p. 48.

15.   Quoted in Phyllis Bentley, *The Brontës and Their World* (New York: Viking, 1969), p. 45.

16.   Elizabeth Gaskell, *The Life of Charlotte Brontë*, with an Introduction by Winifred Gerin (London and New York: Dent & Dutton, 1974), p. 60.

17.   "She is (as she calls herself) *undeveloped*; thin and more than half a head shorter than I . . ." In a letter to Catherine Winkworth, 25 August 1850, *SHBLL*, vol. 3, p. 142.

18.   Gaskell observes that "as her limbs and head were in just proportion to the slight, fragile body, no word in ever so slight *a* degree suggestive of deformity could properly be applied to her" (*Life*, p. 60).

19.   *SHBLL*, vol. 4, p. 181.

20.   Bessie adds that "gentility" is as much as she had expected to see in Jane's person, since "you were no beauty as a child" (p. 123).

21.   See the discussion in Rebecca Fraser, *The Brontës: Charlotte Brontë and Her Family* (New York: Fawcett Columbine, 1988), pp. 36–38.

22.   Ibid., pp. 27–28.

23.   *SHBLL*, vol. 1, p. 92.

24.   Ibid.

25.   Ibid., vol. 1, p. 94.

26.   Gaskell, *Life*, p. 147.

27.   *SHBLL*, vol. 3, p. 142.

28.   Gaskell, *Life*, p. 380.

29.   Ibid., p. 61.

30.   Charlotte Brontë, *Five Novelettes*, transcribed from the original manuscripts and ed. Winifred Gerin (London: Folio Press, 1971), p. 15.

31.   Ibid., p. 99. (*Julia* was written in 1837).

32.   Ibid., p. 158.

33.   Charlotte Brontë, *An Edition of the Early Writings of Charlotte Brontë*, ed. Christine Alexander (Oxford, U.K., and New York: Published for the Shakespeare Head Press by B. Blackwell, 1987), p. 209.

34.   "Henry Hastings," in *Five Novelettes*, ed. Winifred Gerin (London: Folio Press, 1971), p. 180.

35.   Ibid., p. 202.

36.   Charlotte Brontë, *The Professor and Emma: A Fragment*, introduction by Anne Smith (London: Dent, 1985), p. xxiii. All subsequent quotations are from this edition.

37.   *The Letters of Mrs Gaskell*, ed. J. A. V. Chapple and Arthur Pollard (Manchester: University of Manchester Press, 1966); quoted in a letter, n. 308.

38.   When Jane explains to Diana, in reference to St. John's proposed missionary marriage, "And I am so plain you see, Di. We should never suit," Diana responds indignantly, "Plain! You? Not at all. You are much too pretty, as well as too good, to be grilled alive in Calcutta" (chap. 35, p. 441).

39.   In their first meeting as strangers on the road (chap. 12, p. 145), and again in their first extended interchange at Thornfield, when Rochester asks Jane whether she thinks him handsome (chap. 14, p. 162).

40.   Charlotte Brontë, *Villette*, ed. Mark Lilly with an Introduction by Tony Tanner (Harmondsworth, England: Penguin, 1979), chap. 33, p. 470.

41.   *The Madwoman in the Attic: The Woman Writer and the Nineteenth-Century Literary Imagination* (New Haven: Yale University Press, 1979) sees the mad Bertha, a prisoner of a patriarchal society, as its central image for the nineteenth-century woman who has to a greater or lesser degree suppressed her own rage and her own best — most honest and most creative — self.

42.   Charlotte Brontë, *Shirley* (Harmondsworth, England: Penguin, 1985), p. 196.

43.   Ibid., p. 193.

44.   *SHBLL*, vol. 4, p. 112.

45.   Chapple and Pollard, *Letters of Mrs. Gaskell*, quoted in n. 195, to John Forster, p. 289.

46.   Fraser, *The Brontës*, p. 483.

47.   Ibid., p. 473.

48.   Ibid., p. 478. In her Introduction, p. xvii, to Brontë's *The Professor and Emma*, Anne Smith expresses the same faith.

49.   Chapple and Pollard, *Letters of Mrs. Gaskell*, p. 496.

50. In an interview with Sir Wemyss Reid; Fraser, *The Brontës*, p. 478.

51. In a letter to Mrs. Humphrey Ward, who was preparing a new edition of the Brontë novels in 1899, in response to her queries about Mrs. Gaskell's claim; quoted in Fraser, *The Brontës*, p. 478.

52. See "Charlotte Brontë's Photograph," *Brontë Society Transactions* (1968), pp. 27–28.

Chapter 5. *George Eliot*

1. The most extreme as well as most trenchant formulation of the twentieth-century feminist indictment of Eliot's typically beautiful "performing" heroine is still Ellen Moers's 1963 assessment: "George Eliot was always concerned with the superior, large-souled woman whose distinction resides not in her deeds but in her capacity to attract attention and arouse admiration." "Performing Heroinism: The Myth of Corinne," in *Literary Woman: The Great Writers* (Garden City, N. Y.: Doubleday & Company, Inc., Anchor Books, 1977), p. 295. Moers singles out Dorothea among Eliot's heroines for particularly harsh criticism as a woman who is "good for nothing *but* to be admired" (p. 296) and whose influence on the later tradition has been damaging. Later feminist critics have been more willing to acknowledge the societal constraints imposed on Dorothea, but still read her story as essentially one of frustrated fulfillment and/or the willed repression of her deepest needs — even if she may in the process hold out a "lifeline" to others. See Gilbert and Gubar, *Madwoman in the Attic*, especially pp. 512–13 and 528. Carolyn Heilbrun is typical of recent feminist criticism in implying a failure of courage on the part of a writer "who did in her life what she could never portray in the lives of her heroines," and only "*allowed* a minor character in *Daniel Deronda* to protest against women's storylessness" (*Writing*, p. 37, my italics). Gillian Beer, in *George Eliot*, Key Women Writers Series, ed. Sue Roe (Bloomington: Indiana University Press, 1986), makes a valiant effort to portray Eliot as a more radical feminist, in both her personal writing and her fiction, than I think the evidence will bear. In my own view, the most balanced assessment of Eliot's complex views on "the women's question" as these are reflected in her actions (or nonactions), her essays, and her fiction, is that in Jennifer Uglow's excellent recent biography, *George Eliot*, in the Virago series (London and New York: Virago/Pantheon, 1987). See particularly chap. 4, " 'George Eliot' and the Woman Question in the 1850's" (pp. 65–81) which stresses ways in which Eliot seeks to qualify more radical feminist attitudes — of both her own age and ours. Uglow, I think, also does well with *Middlemarch* (chap. 12, "Middlemarch: Against Simplicity," pp. 193–216), where she emphasizes

Dorothea's "female power" and the way the ending suggests a potential for action if not the realization.

2.   George Eliot, *Middlemarch*, ed. W. J. Harvey (Harmondsworth, England: Penguin, 1965), chap. 1, p. 29. All subsequent quotations are from this edition.

3.   In a letter to the Brays, written on 12 March 1853 (shortly after the collapse of her romantic relationship with Herbert Spenser and on the eve of the all-important one with George Lewes, Marian Evans had written to the Brays, "Villette — Villette — have you read it?" (Haight, *Letters*, vol. 2, p. 92). In a letter of the previous week, written with Lewes's account of his meeting with Brontë fresh in her mind, she observed that while the woman herself might be "a little, plain, provincial, sickly-looking old maid, yet what passion, what fire in her!" (vol. 2, p. 91). At a key moment in her own life, then, just as she was changing in her own person from a "hideous hag" to a beautiful, loved woman, Eliot identified with the sexual passion that, however thwarted or repressed, comes through so strongly in Lucy Snowe. On their wedding journey to the continent she and Lewes visited Brussels, which she makes a point of identifying as the "Labassecour" of *Villette*.

4.   "But what a voice! It was like the voice of a soul that had once lived in an Aeolian harp. This must be one of Nature's inconsistencies. There could be no sort of passion in a girl who would marry Casaubon" (chap. 9, p. 105).

5.   Haight, *Letters*, vol. 1, p. 167 (16 February 1852).

6.   Ibid., vol. 2, p. 25 (5 May 1852).

7.   Ibid., vol. 2, p. 29 (27 May 1852).

8.   Ibid., vol. 2, p. 251 ("Recollections of Ilfracombe").

9.   For Milly, see "Amos Barton," in *Scenes of Clerical Life*, ed. David Lodge (Harmondsworth, England: Penguin, 1973), p. 54. For Janet Dempster, see "Janet's Repentance," ibid., p. 284.

10.   For Nancy Lammeter, see *Silas Marner: The Weaver of Raveloe*, ed. with an Introduction by Q. D. Leavis (London & N.Y.: Penguin, 1985), p. 143.

11.   Eliot, *Adam Bede*, ed. Stephen Gill (Harmondsworth, England: Penguin, 1980), p. 128. All subsequent quotations are from this edition.

12.   *The Mill on the Floss*, ed. with an Introduction and notes by A. S. Byatt (Harmondsworth, England: Penguin, 1979), bk. 1, chap. 7, pp. 116–17. All subsequent quotations are from this edition.

13.   Interestingly, such a disequilibrium is not present in the Parthenon sculpture itself, where the heads of *both* figures are missing. Eliot transforms the

image in her own presentation to create a relation (whether negative or positive in its implications) between figures of differing strengths.

14.   In a letter to her friend and former teacher, Maria Lewis, written in 1840, she says, "You must know I have had bestowed on me [by another close friend and schoolmate, Patty Jackson] the very pretty cognomen of Clematis, which in Floral language, means Mental Beauty. I cannot find it in my heart to refuse it, though like many other appellations it has rather the appearance of a satire than a compliment" (Haight, *Letters*, vol. 1, p. 67).

15.   See Moers, "Performing Heroinism," p. 297.

16.   George Eliot, *Daniel Deronda*, ed. with an Introduction by Barbara Hardy (London and New York: Viking-Penguin, 1986), p. 35. All subsequent quotations are from this edition.

17.   "If anyone objected to the turn of her nose or the form of her neck and chin, she had not the sense that she could presently show her power of attainment in these branches of feminine perfection." Ibid., chap. 23, p. 294.

18.   *George Eliot's Life as Related in Her Letters and Journals.* "Arranged and Edited by Her Husband, J. W. Cross," 3 vols. (New York: Harper & Brothers, 1885), vol. 3, pp. 59–60.

19.   Henry James, *Selected Letters*, ed. Leon Edel (Cambridge, Mass.: Belknap Press of Harvard University Press, 1987), p. 35.

20.   See also John Fiske's detailed account to his wife in a letter of 23 November 1873: "Well, what do I think of her? She is not a "fright" by any means. She is a plain-looking woman, but I think not especially homely." Having inventoried her features (good nose, expressive eyes, large mouth, etc.), he concludes: "I never saw such a woman. There is nothing a bit masculine about her; she is thoroughly feminine and looks and acts as if she were fit for nothing but to mother babies. But she has a power of *stating* an argument equal to any man; equal I do say, I never have seen any . . . who could state a case equal to her" (Haight, *Letters*, vol. 5, pp. 436–69). See also Bret Hart's account, in a letter of January 1880: "I was very pleasantly disappointed in her appearance, having heard so much of the plainness of her features. And I found them only strong, intellectual, and *noble* — indeed, I have seldom seen a grander face. . . . It expresses elevation of thought, kindness, power, and *humour* (Haight, *Letters*, vol. 7, p. 241).

21.   As early as the writing of *Adam Bede*, when Eliot is still struggling with the beauty question, attempting intermittently to "write off" the effect of Hetty's all-too-seductive beauty, and, in a flourishing authorial aside, tells the reader she can't afford to fill the pages of her work with portraits of such rar-

ities as "sublimely beautiful women," her announced dedication to a realistic aesthetic and a true-to-life homeliness concludes with the fine (and quintessentially Eliot) affirmation that "human feeling is like the mighty rivers that bless the earth: it does not wait for beauty — it flows with resistless force *and brings beauty with it*" (chap. 17, p. 224, my italics).

Chapter 6. *Two Mastectomy Narratives*

1. "A Mastectomy at the hands of Baron Larrey, Napoleon's famous army surgeon: 30 September 1811, Letter (Berg) to Esther Burney, 22 March–June 1812," in Fanny Burney, *Selected Letters and Journals*, ed. Joyce Hemlowe (Oxford: Clarendon Press, 1986), pp. 127–40. All subsequent quotations are from this edition.

2. Julia Epstein, "Writing the Unspeakable: Fanny Burney's Mastectomy and the Fictive Body," *Representations* 16 (Fall 1986), pp. 131–66. Reprinted as a chapter in Epstein's *The Iron Pen: Fanny Burney and the Politics of Women's Writing* (Madison: University of Wisconsin Press, 1989).

3. A letter of 7 March 1795, to Mrs Waddington, in Hemlowe, *Selected Letters and Journals*, p. 33.

4. Richard Selzer, *Raising the Dead: A Doctor's Encounter with His Own Mortality* (New York: Viking-Whittle, 1993), p. 5.

5. Betty Rollins, *First, You Cry* (1976; New York: Signet, New American Library, 1977), p. 146.

6. Ronald Melzack, "Phantom Limbs," *Scientific American* (April, 1992), p. 123.

7. Susan Love, whose authoritative and most helpful work, *Dr. Susan Love's Breast Book*, with Karen Lindsey, (Reading, Mass.: Addison Wesley Publishing Company, Inc., 1990), is an exception here. She does not go into the issue in depth, but Love does make the distinction between how the reconstructed breast looks on the outside (to others) and how it feels on the inside (to the woman herself). Though, speaking from my own experience, I might be more affirmative than she is here, the important thing is that she does make the distinction. Noting that "it's important to understand [the] limits [of reconstructive breast surgery] before you decide to have it done," Love goes on to say: "What's constructed is *not* a real breast. When it's well done, it will *look* real, but it will never have full sensation, as a breast does. It's more like a prosthesis attached to your chest. Any surgeon who tells you, 'We're going to take off your breast and give you a new one, and it'll be as good as new' is either

stupid or dishonest. Sometimes they'll tell you that the new breast 'feels normal' — at best, a half-truth. It will feel normal to the hand that's touching it, but it will have little feeling itself. It will never feel completely normal to you" (p. 350).

Chapter 7. *The Beauty of Age*

1. Germaine Greer, *The Change: Women, Aging and the Menopause* (New York: Knopf, 1992). All subsequent quotations are from this edition.

2. See also Carolyn Heilbrun's essay, "Coming of Age," *New York Woman* (Feb., 1991), in which she describes women finally being able to move, with age, into a world where "we live by what we do, not by how we look or who looks at us. . . . As real as the men in the world we formerly occupied, we will take the reality we recognized only in them and claim it for ourselves" (p. 58). In *Writing Women's Lives* Heilbrun speaks with similar admiration for women who allow themselves in their later years to "dissociate their personhood from their feminine appeal," to become overweight, disheveled, and generally show a gutsy disregard for their appearances, as if only then could they say to men, "I do not want to attract you. I want to enjoy myself as a human being" (pp. 54–55).

3. Betty Friedan, *The Fountain of Age* (New York: Simon & Schuster, 1993), p. 164. Friedan's message — that we consider what age brings rather than what it takes away (for both sexes) — is one I find wonderfully exhilarating. I only wish she had included in her model the realm of appearances, as an area in which age makes its own contribution rather than one which is best laid aside.

4. Doris Grumbach, "Coming into the End Zone," pp. 75–87, in *Minding the Body: Women Writers on Body and Soul*, ed. with an Introduction by Patricia Foster (New York: Doubleday & Company, Inc., 1994), p. 77. In this honest and affecting meditation (a series of diary entries written between her seventieth and seventy-first birthdays), Grumbach moves toward a state of mind in which she becomes not only more accepting of her age but more able to relish its special pleasures. In the concluding entry, written on her seventy-first birthday, she speaks of the pleasure of an early-morning swim, in which she conquered the 60-degree temperature of the water "by thinking it was not as cold as I expected it to be" (p. 86). The concluding lines of the piece — "Unlike Anna Pavlova, I have no immediate use for a swan costume. I am ready to begin the end" — suggest to me not a repudiation of but an enjoyment in her body, unmasked, as it is.

5.   See Greer, *The Change*, pp. 28–30. To this brief list I might add the three heroines of Mary Gordon's more recent novel, *The Rest of Life: Three Novellas* (Harmondsworth, England: Penguin, 1993).

6.   Margaret Drabble, *The Realms of Gold* (New York: Knopf, 1975), pp. 92–93.

7.   Mary Meigs, *In the Company of Strangers* (Vancouver: Talonbooks, 1991), p. 10.

Index

Adam Bede (Eliot), Hetty Sorrel
heroine-portraiture in, 137–38,
143–44, 145
Aging, beauty and: menopause, 182–
85; older-women heroines, 189–
90; *Strangers in Good Company*
(film), 190–203
Andersen, Hans Christian, "becoming beautiful" motif in *The Ugly
Duckling*, 88–90
Anorexia, 24–25
Appearances: and defining beauty as
the face of love, 10–12; physical
features of heroes and heroines,
45–46; women's concern for, 15–
17, 26–28
Ariosto, Ludovico, 38
Ashworth (Brontë), 108
As You Like It (Shakespeare),
heroine-portraiture in, 31–32
Austen, Jane: Anne Elliot heroine-
portraiture in *Persuasion*, 83–86;
Elizabeth Bennet heroine-
portraiture in *Pride and Prejudice*,
69–71, 73, 74; Fanny Price
heroine-portraiture in *Mansfield
Park*, 82–83; "pretty" heroines
and "handsome" women, 71–73,
74, 82–83

*B*agehot, Walter, 100–101
Beauty: and aging, 181–203; beauty
question comparison between
Eliot and Brontë, 131–33;
"becoming beautiful" motif in
women's fiction, 81–90; and child-

hood ugliness, 6–10, 12, 98–99;
child's knowledge of her, 11;
clothing and heroine's, 137–38,
139, 143, 146; defining beauty as
the face of love, 10–12; and early
childhood memories, 1–7; fairness
of beauty concept, 58–67; and
female ugliness, 43–44, 59–67,
71, 80, 95–96, 136–37, 144–45; as
a gift concept, 90–94; hand and
arm symbolism and, 133–34, 138–
40, 141–42, 145; handsomeness
vs., 46–47; heroines' beauty in
fairy tales, 78–80; heroines of
"difficult" beauty, 70–71, 75–78,
106, 110, 137–38, 148–49; illness
and the lack of, 96–97; individual's perception of, 11–12; for a
man's love, 12–13; and plainness,
57, 58, 99–103, 107; postindustrial
age, 46; and presence, 148–49;
"pretty" heroines vs. "handsome"
women, 71–73, 74, 82–83; self-
assertion and, 83; small and plain
heroines, 99–103, 106–9, 110–16;
thinness and, 15
Beauty Myth, The (Wolf), 15, 24–25
Bell, Currer *see* Brontë, Charlotte
Bettelheim, Bruno, 78–79
Biopsies, 168
Bleak House (Dickens), 66
Bluest Eye, The (Morrison), 203;
"black is beautiful," 15; childhood
ugliness in, 7–10, 12
Book of the Courtier, The (Castiglione), 10–11

Breast development, 13–14
Breast reconstruction, 170, 176–80
Breast removal: without anesthesia,
    151, 152. *See also* Mastectomy
    narratives
Brontë, Charlotte: beauty question
    comparison between Eliot and,
    131–33; childhood, 103; Frances
    Henri heroine-portraiture in *The
    Professor* and *Emma: A Fragment*,
    109–10, 118–19; heroines of "dif-
    ficult" beauty, 75, 110; lack of
    beauty, 95, 96; marriage, 96, 124–
    25; photographic image of, 126–
    27; Richmond portrait of, 97; sex-
    ual paradise symbolism in *Shirley*,
    123–24; shrinking manner, 104–6;
    small and plain heroines, 75, 99–
    103, 106–9, 110–16; smallness of,
    102, 103–4. *See also Jane Eyre*;
    Villette
Brownmiller, Susan, 13–15
Burke, Edmund, 78
Burney, Esther, 151–52, 153
Burney, Fanny: beauty contrast
    between heroine and rival in, 74–
    75; fairness of beauty concept in
    Camilla, 58–67; mastectomy nar-
    rative, 151–67

Camilla (Burney): beauty contrast
    between heroine and rival in, 74–
    75; disfigured heroine in, 58–67,
    156, 157
Captain Henry Hastings (Brontë), 108
Castiglione, Baldesar, 10–11
*Change: Women, Aging, and the Meno-
    pause, The* (Greer), 182–85
Chaucer, Geoffrey, 46
Children: adolescent girls, 23–24;
    childhood curiosity, 19; childhood
    "dress-up" play, 181–82; child-
    hood reminiscences, 1–7; child-
    hood ugliness, 7–10, 12, 98–99;
    child's knowledge of her beauty,
    11
Cinderella, 78–80
*Clarissa: Or the History of a Young
    Lady* (Richardson), heroine-
    portraiture in, 51–54

Cleopatra, 31, 117, 131–33, 190
Clinique Turnaround Cream, 188
Clitoral orgasm, 14
Cœlebs in Search of a Wife (More), 67
Colby, Alice, 43
"Coming into the End Zone"
    (Grumbach), 187–88
Countenance, beauty of, 67–68, 82,
    106
"Criticism of Female Beauty"
    (Hunt), 37
Cross, John, 146
Curiosity, childhood, 19

Daniel Deronda (Eliot): Gwendolyn
    Harleth heroine-portraiture in,
    145–46; relation between beauty
    and presence in, 148–49
d'Arblay, Count, 151, 154, 155, 159,
    160
Deerbrook (Martineau), 75
Demers, Gloria, 192
de Narbonne, M., 155
Dickens, Charles, 66
Donne, John, 39, 42–43, 67
Drabble, Margaret, 189, 203; Sarah
    heroine-portraiture in *A Summer
    Bird-Cage*, 90–94
Dr. Thorne (Trollope), 76
Dubois, M., 154, 158–59, 162, 164

Eliot, George: Dorothea Brooke
    heroine-portraiture in *Middle-
    march*, 129–36, 137, 141–42, 143,
    147–48, 149; Gwendolyn Harleth
    heroine-portraiture in *Daniel
    Deronda*, 145–46; heroines of "dif-
    ficult" beauty, 75, 137–38, 148–
    49; Hetty Sorrel heroine-
    portraiture in *Adam Bede*, 137–38,
    143–44, 145; lack of beauty, 95–
    96, 136–37; Maggie Tulliver
    heroine-portraiture in *The Mill on
    the Floss*, 138–41; marriage, 146;
    relationship with George Lewes,
    128, 136, 137, 141, 142, 147
Emma (Austen), 72–73
Epstein, Julia, 152
Eros, 38
Eroticism, 38–39

Eustace Diamonds, The (Trollope), 76
Evans, Marian *see* Eliot, George
Expression, countenance and, 67–68

Fairy tales: "becoming beautiful"
motif in *The Ugly Duckling*, 88–
90; heroines' beauty in, 78–80
Female body: breast development,
13–14; breast reconstruction, 176–
80; breast removal without anesthesia, 151, 152; developing, 13–
14; differences between male and
female genitalia, 21; hand and arm
symbolism, 133–34, 138–40, 141–
42, 145; mammography, 167–68;
menopause, 182–85; objectified in
literature, 31; physical features of
heroes and heroines, 45–46;
woman's genitalia in twelfth-
century French literature, 43
Feminine vanity, 15
Femininity (Brownmiller), 13–15
Feminism: feminist movement of the
1960s, 14; value of appearances
and, 16–17
Fielding, Henry, 45, 48
First You Cry (Rollins), 172, 173,
176
French romances, twelfth-century,
41–46
Freud, Sigmund, 57; eroticism, 38–
39; notion of scopophilia, 19–21,
194
Friedan, Betty, 24, 25, 185

Gaskell, Elizabeth, 75, 110; biog-
raphy of Charlotte Brontë, 97,
105–6, 124, 125; Molly Gibson
heroine-portraiture in *Wives and
Daughters*, 86–88
Gazes, masculine, 15–16, 19–22, 30,
31, 38, 174; gaze of a man's body,
44–45
Geoffrey of Vinsauf, 42
Gilbert, Sandra M., 122–23
Gilbert, W. S., 42
Gordimer, Nadine, 56
Greer, Germaine, 182–85
Grumbach, Doris, 187–88
Gubar, Susan, 122–23

Handsomeness: beauty vs., 46–47;
"pretty" heroines vs. "handsome"
women, 71–73, 74, 82–83
Hebraic poetry, 40–41
Heger, M., 109, 116
Heilbrun, Carolyn G., 16–17, 204
Helen of Troy, 31
Herbert, George, 118
Hero and Leander (Marlowe), 44–45
Heroine-portraiture: feminine con-
vention of, 58–76; patriarchal
convention of, 31–54
Homosexual love, 45
House, symbolism in women's fic-
tion, 118–24
Humbert, Humbert, 71
Hunt, Leigh, 37

Illness: and the lack of beauty, 96–
97; smallpox and ugliness, 59–60
Immured maiden, the, 62–63
Inchbald, Elizabeth, 68–69
In the Company of Strangers (Meigs),
192, 196, 197, 199, 201–2
Ivanhoe (Scott), Rebecca-Rowena
heroine-portraiture in, 32–37, 38,
39–40, 48

James, Henry, 146–47
Jane Eyre (Brontë): xii; childhood
ugliness in, 98–99; concept of
beauty and plainness in, 57, 58,
99–102; heroine of "difficult"
beauty in, 110; sexual paradise
symbolism in, 119–20; small and
plain heroine in, 99–103, 107, 108,
110–16
Johnson, Samuel, 60, 67, 71
Joseph Andrews (Fielding), 45
Joyce, James, 49–50
Julia (Brontë), 107
Juvenilian novelettes, 107–8

Kempley, Rita, 191

Laocoön, The (G. Lessing), 37
Larrey, Dr.: letter to Fanny Burney,
159–60; relationship with patient
Fanny Burney, 155–56, 157–58,
165, 166

Lawrence, D. H., 58
Lesbianism, 199–201
Lessing, Doris, 56, 189
Lessing, Gotthold, 37–38
Lewes, George, relationship with
    George Eliot, 128, 136, 137, 141,
    142, 147
Life and Opinions of Tristram Shandy,
    The (Sterne), 48
Literature: female novelists heroine-
    portraiture portrayal in women's
    fiction, 55–94; male novelists
    heroine-portraiture portrayal in
    Western, 31–54; twelfth-century
    French, 41–46
Lolita (Nabokov), heroine-
    portraiture in, 50–51, 71
"Loves Progress" (Donne), 42–43
Lumpectomy, 163

Madwoman in the Attic, The (Gil-
    bert and Gubar), 122–23
Male body: differences between male
    and female genitalia, 21; gaze of a
    man's body, 44–45; male ejacula-
    tion, 14; the male gaze, 15–16, 19–
    22, 30, 31, 38, 174; physical fea-
    tures of heroes and heroines, 45–
    46; scopophilia, 19–20
Male/female relations, doctor patient
    relationship in, 155–67
Male novelists: heroine-portraiture
    portrayal in Western literature,
    31–54; portrayal of heroines as
    "difficult" beauties, 76–77
Mammography, 167–68
Mann, Delbert, 35
Mansfield Park (Austen): Fanny Price
    heroine-portraiture in, 82–83;
    "ugly duckling" heroine in,
    71–72
Marlowe, Christopher, 44–45
Marriageable women, 96
Martineau, Harriet, 75, 102
Marty (film), 35
Maslin, Janet, 191
Mastectomy narratives: of Fanny
    Burney, 151–67; of Ellen Zetzel
    Lambert, 167–80
Matthew of Vendôme, 43–44, 46

Meigs, Mary, In the Company of
    Strangers, 192, 193, 196, 197, 199,
    201–2
Melzack, Ronald, 178, 179
Menopause, 182–85
Middlemarch (Eliot), Dorothea
    Brooke heroine-portraiture in,
    129–36, 137, 141–42, 143, 147–
    48, 149
Mill on the Floss, The (Eliot), Maggie
    Tulliver heroine-portraiture in,
    138–41
Milton, John, 118
Mina Laury (Brontë), 107–8
More, Hannah, 67
Morrison, Toni, 7–10, 12, 15, 203

Nabokov, Vladimir, 50–51, 71
Nicholls, Rev. Arthur, marriage
    to Charlotte Brontë, 96, 124,
    125–26
North and South (Gaskell), 75
Northanger Abbey (Austen), 71
Nussey, Ellen, 97, 104–5, 124, 125

Older sisters, "pretty" heroines
    and, 71–72
Older-women heroines, 189–90
Oliphant, Margaret, 75
Orgasm, clitoral, 14
Ozick, Cynthia, 56

Pamela: Or Virtue Rewarded (Rich-
    ardson), 73–74
Paradise, sexual symbolism in wom-
    en's fiction, 118–24
Patriarchal society: language and
    women's speech within a, 15;
    patriarchal convention of heroine-
    portraiture, 31–54
"Peep into a Picture-Book, A," 107
Perrault, Charles, 79
Persuasion (Austen), 72; Anne Elliot
    heroine-portraiture in, 83–86
Petrarch, 37
"Phantom limb" phenomenon, 178–
    79
Philosophical Inquiry into the Sublime
    and the Beautiful, A (Burke), 78
Physiognomy, 99

Pickering, Sir George White, 96
Poetria Nova (Geoffrey of Vinsauf), 42
Portrait of the Artist (Joyce), heroine-portraiture in, 49–50
Post-menopausal women, 184–85
Pride and Prejudice (Austen), Elizabeth Bennet heroine-portraiture in, 69–71, 73, 74
Professor and Emma: A Fragment, The (Brontë), 125; Frances Henri heroine-portraiture in, 109–10, 118–19
Proust, Marcel, 37

Quarterly Review, 99

Raising the Dead (Selzer), 166
Rambler, The (Johnson), 60
Rape, 14; poem about, 43
Realms of Gold, The (Drabble), 189, 203
Recollections (Eliot), 137
Richardson, Samuel: heroine-portraiture in *Clarissa*, 51–54; heroine-portraiture in *Pamela*, 73–74
Rigby, Elizabeth, review of *Jane Eyre*, 99–100
Rime (Petrarch), 37
Rollins, Betty, 172, 173, 176
Romance of the Rose (Chaucer), 46
Room of One's Own, A (Woolf), 56

Scenes of Clerical Life (Eliot), 137
Scopophilia, 19–20, 194
Scott, Cynthia, 192, 196–97
Scott, Sir Walter, Rebecca-Rowena heroine-portraiture in *Ivanhoe*, 32–37, 38, 39–40, 48
Self-assertion, beauty and, 83
Self-esteem, 27
Selzer, Richard, 165–66
Sex: Cleopatra's sexuality, 117, 131–33; sexual paradise symbolism in women's fiction, 118–24; and women's fiction, 57
Shakespeare, William 31–32, 55, 190
Shirley (Brontë), 115; sexual paradise symbolism in, 123–24

Siblings, older sisters and "pretty" heroines, 71–72
Silas Marner: The Weaver of Raveloe (Eliot), 137
Simple Story, A (Inchbald), heroine-portraiture in, 68–69
Skin cream advertisers, 188
Small, and plain heroines, 99–103, 106–9, 110–16
Smallpox, ugliness and, 59–60
Song of Songs, The, 40–41
Spectator essays, 64
Spencer, Herbert, 136
Sterne, Laurence, 48–49
Stout women, 108
Strangers in Good Company (film), 190–203
Summer Before the Dark, The (D. Lessing), 189
Summer Bird-Cage, A (Drabble), Sarah heroine-portraiture in, 90–94, 189

Tesher, Dr., 171, 175
Thackeray, William Makepeace, 48
Thinness: anorexia, 24–25; and beauty, 15
"To His Mistress Going to Bed" (Donne), 39
Trollope, Anthony, portrayal of heroines as "difficult" beauties, 76–77

Ugliness: childhood, 6–10, 12, 98–99; female, 43–44, 59–67, 71, 80, 95–96, 136–37, 144–45; smallpox and, 58–60; "ugly duckling" heroine, 71
Ugly Duckling, The (Andersen), "becoming beautiful" motif in the, 88–90

Villette (Brontë), 109; comparison to Eliot's *Middlemarch*, 131–33; Lucy Snow heroine-portraiture in, 115, 116–18; sexual paradise symbolism in, 120–22

Walt Disney, 79
Wanderer, The (Burney), 151

Warden, The (Trollope), "difficult" beauty heroine in, 76–77

Watsons, The (Austen), 72

West Side Story, xi

Wives and Daughters (Gaskell), Molly Gibson heroine-portraiture in, 86–88

Wolf, Naomi, 14–15, 24–25, 28–29

Wollstonecraft, Mary, 14, 15

Women novelists, 55–58; beauty as a gift concept in women's fiction, 90–94; "becoming beautiful" motif in women's fiction, 81–90; feminine convention of heroine-portraiture, 58–76; feminist criticism of *Cinderella*, 78–80; invention of heroines of "difficult" beauty, 70–71, 75–76, 77–78. *See also* Brontë, Charlotte; Eliot, George

Women's movement: of the 1960s, 14, 23

Woolf, Virginia, 56

Writing a Woman's Life (Heilbrun), 16–17

Zeuxis, 31